CRASH COURSE

Self-Assessment
IN Medicine
AND Surgery

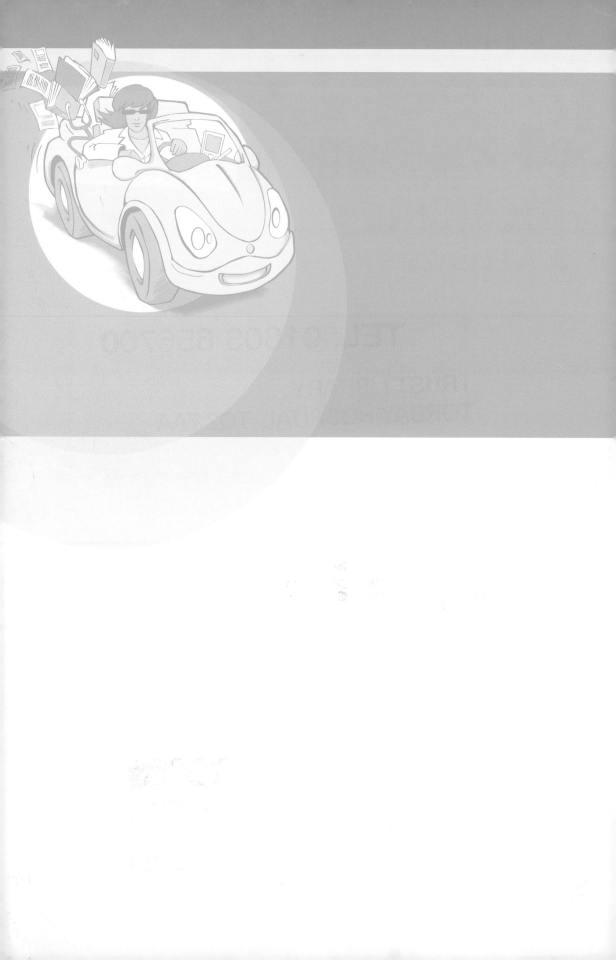

CRASH COURSE

Self-Assessment IN Medicine AND Surgery

Series editor
Daniel Horton-Szar
BSc (Hons), MBBS (Hons), MRCGP
General Practitioner,
Northgate Medical Practice,
Canterbury, UK

Faculty advisor (Medicine)
Anne Ballinger
MD, MRCP
Consultant Gastroenterologist
and General Physician Queen
Elizabeth the Queen Mother
Hospital, Margate, Kent, UK

Faculty advisor (Surgery)
Marc Gladman
PhD, MRCOG, FRCS (Gen Surg)
Centre for Academic Surgery,
Barts and The London School of
Medicine & Dentistry, University
of London, London, UK

Neel Sharma
BSc (Hons), MBChB
Foundation Year One Doctor,
The Royal London Hospital,
Barts and the London NHS Trust, London, UK

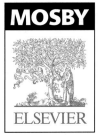

MOSBY

ELSEVIER

Edinburgh • London • New York • Oxford • Philadelphia • St Louis • Sydney • Toronto 2009

MOSBY
ELSEVIER

Commissioning Editor:	*Alison Taylor*
Development Editor:	*Fiona Conn*
Project Manager:	*Elouise Ball*
Page design:	*Sarah Russell*
Icon illustrations:	*Geo Parkin*
Cover design:	*Stewart Larking*

First edition 2009

ISBN: 978-0-7234-3510-5

British Library Cataloguing in Publication Data
A catalogue record for this book is available from the British Library

Library of Congress Cataloging in Publication Data
A catalog record for this book is available from the Library of Congress

Note
Knowledge and best practice in this field are constantly changing. As new research and experience broaden our knowledge, changes in practice, treatment and drug therapy may become necessary or appropriate. Readers are advised to check the most current information provided (i) on procedures featured or (ii) by the manufacturer of each product to be administered, to verify the recommended dose or formula, the method and duration of administration, and contraindications. It is the responsibility of the practitioner, relying on their own experience and knowledge of the patient, to make diagnoses, to determine dosages and the best treatment for each individual patient, and to take all appropriate safety precautions. To the fullest extent of the law, neither the Publisher nor the Editors/Authors assumes any liability for any injury and/or damage to persons or property arising out or related to any use of the material contained in this book.

The Publisher

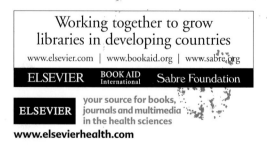

The publisher's policy is to use **paper manufactured from sustainable forests**

Printed in China

As a recent medical graduate I understand all too well the pressures faced during medical school. Lectures, tutorials, never ending ward rounds, outpatient clinics, course work assignments and, of course, let us not forget the gruelling end-of-year exams. Trying to retain, and more importantly, understand all the common (and not so common) clinical diseases and presentations truly seems an impossible task.

With the advent of the Universities Medical Assessment Partnership (UMAP) there has now been a move away from testing specific clinical facts to an assessment focused on preparing yourself as a foundation doctor and the knowledge such a trainee needs on a day to day basis. Currently fourteen UK medical schools are part of UMAP and their exams now require candidates to decide for example what would be the most appropriate initial investigation or what management plan they would instigate first when faced with a clinical problem. Hardly an easy task based on the little experience one gains as an undergraduate in such decisions.

This self-assessment book is designed to help students tackle both the new form of assessment as well as the traditional style of examination. Questions covering all common medical and surgical presentations are included as MCQ and EMQ formats with relevant, concise explanations as answers.

I sincerely hope that this book is of use in preparing for your forthcoming examinations and wish you all the success in your future medical careers.

Neel Sharma

"Education and work are the levers to uplift a people. Work alone will not do it unless inspired by the right ideals and guided by intelligence."

W E B Du Bois 1868–1963

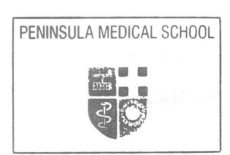

PENINSULA MEDICAL SCHOOL

Medicine never stands still, and the work of keeping this series relevant for today's students is an ongoing process. These new self-assessment titles build upon the success of the preceding books and represent a great deal of brand new exam preparation material, keeping the series up to date with the latest examination formats that face today's medical students.

As always, we listen to feedback from the thousands of students who use the *Crash Course* revision titles, and have gathered information on current examination practices from medical schools across the UK. This self-assessment book provides a comprehensive range of questions covering the medical and surgical curricula, divided into chapters by topic to help you focus your revision. Questions cover both the common Single Best Answer (SBA) and Extended Matching Question (EMQ) formats.

Despite fully revising the series on a regular basis, and adding new titles, we hold fast to the principles on which we first developed the series: *Crash Course* will always bring you all the information you need to revise in compact, manageable volumes that integrate pathology and therapeutics with best clinical practice, and now we are expanding our range of self-assessment titles. The books still maintain the balance between clarity and conciseness, and providing sufficient depth for those aiming at distinction. The authors are junior doctors who have recent experience of the exams you are now facing, and the accuracy of the material is checked by senior clinicians and faculty members from across the UK.

I wish you all the best for your future careers!

Dan Horton-Szar
Series Editor

Acknowledgements

I would like to acknowledge Dr Anne Ballinger and Mr Marc Gladman for their most valuable input during the development of this volume.

*I would like to dedicate this book to my parents,
Ravi and Anita, and my sister Ravnita.
Without their continued support and
encouragement none of this would
have been truly possible.*

Contents

Normal values xiii

QUESTIONS

Section 1 Medicine. 1

1. Rheumatology. 3
2. Respiratory medicine. 9
3. Endocrinology and diabetes 17
4. Renal medicine 27
5. Neurology. 33
6. Haematology 45
7. Cardiovascular medicine 53
8. Gastroenterology and hepatobiliary medicine 61

Section 2 Surgery 71

9. Surgical emergencies. 73
10. Hernia. 77
11. Vascular surgery 79
12. Breast disease 83
13. Orthopaedics 87
14. Ear, nose and throat. 91
15. Trauma 95
16. Urology. 99
17. Perioperative care 103
18. Gastrointestinal surgery 105

ANSWERS

Section 3 Medicine. 111

1. Rheumatology. 113
2. Respiratory medicine. 115
3. Endocrinology and diabetes 119
4. Renal medicine 123
5. Neurology. 125
6. Haematology 129
7. Cardiovascular medicine 133
8. Gastroenterology and hepatobiliary medicine 135

Section 4 Surgery 139

9. Surgical emergencies. 141
10. Hernia. 143
11. Vascular surgery 145
12. Breast disease 147
13. Orthopaedics 149
14. Ear, nose and throat 151
15. Trauma 153
16. Urology. 155
17. Perioperative care 157
18. Gastrointestinal surgery 159

Index 161

Normal values

HAEMATOLOGY

Haemoglobin
Male	13.5–17.7 g/dL
Female	11.5–16.5 g/dL

Mean corpuscular haemoglobin (MCH)	27–32 pg
Mean corpuscular haemoglobin concentration (MCHC)	32–36 g/dL
Mean corpuscular volume (MCV)	80–96 fL

Packed cell volume (PCV)
Male	0.40–0.54 L/L
Female	0.37–0.47 L/L
White blood count (WBC)	4–11 × 10^9/L
Basophil granulocytes	<0.01–0.1 × 10^9/L
Eosinophil granulocytes	0.04–0.4 × 10^9/L
Lymphocytes	1.5–4.0 × 10^9/L
Monocytes	0.2–0.8 × 10^9/L
Neutrophil granulocytes	2.0–7.5 × 10^9/L
Platelet count	150–400 × 10^9/L
Serum B_{12}	160–925 ng/L (150–675 pmol/L)
Serum folate	2.9–18 µg/L (3.6–63 nmol/L)
Red cell folate	149–640 µg/L

Red cell mass
Male	25–35 mL/kg
Female	20–30 mL/kg
Reticulocyte count	0.5–2.5% of red cells (50–100 × 10^9/L)
Erythrocyte sedimentation rate (ESR)	<20 mm in 1 hour

COAGULATION

Bleeding time (Ivy method)	3–9 min
Activated partial thromboplastin time (APTT)	23–31 s
Prothrombin time	12–16 s
International Normalized Ratio (INR)	1.0–1.3
D-dimer	<500 ng/mL

LIPIDS AND LIPOPROTEINS

Cholesterol	3.5–6.5 mmol/L (ideal <5.2 mmol/L)

HDL cholesterol
Male	0.8–1.8 mmol/L
Female	1.0–2.3 mmol/L
LDL cholesterol	<4.0 mmol/L

Triglycerides
Male	0.70–2.1 mmol/L
Female	0.50–1.70 mmol/L

BIOCHEMISTRY (SERUM/PLASMA)

Alanine aminotransferase (ALT)	5–40 U/L
Albumin	35–50 g/L
Alkaline phosphatase	39–117 U/L
Amylase	25–125 U/L
Aspartate aminotransferase (AST)	12–40 U/L
Bicarbonate	22–30 mmol/L
Bilirubin	<17 µmol/L (0.3–1.5 mg/dL)
Calcium	2.20–2.67 mmol/L (8.5–10.5 mg/dL)
Chloride	98–106 mmol/L
C-reactive protein	<10 mg/L
Creatinine	79–118 µmol/L (0.6–1.5 mg/dL)

Creatine kinase (CPK)
Female	24–170 U/L
Male	24–195 U/L
CK–MB fraction	<25 U/L (<60% of total activity)

Ferritin
Female	6–100 µg/L
Male	20–260 µg/L
Postmenopausal	12–230 µg/L
α-Fetoprotein	<10 kU/L
Glucose (fasting)	4.5–5.6 mmol/L (70–110 mg/dL)

γ-Glutamyl transpeptidase (γ-GT)
Male	11–58 U/L
Female	7–32 U/L
Glycosylated (glycated) haemoglobin (HbA_{1c})	3.7–5.1%
Iron	13–32 µmol/L (50–150 µg/dL)
Iron-binding capacity (total) (TIBC)	42–80 µmol/L (250–410 µg/dL)
Magnesium	0.7–1.1 mmol/L
Osmolality	275–295 mOsm/kg
Phosphate	0.8–1.5 mmol/L
Potassium	3.5–5.0 mmol/L
Prostate-specific antigen (PSA)	≤4.0 µg/L
Protein (total)	62–77 g/L
Sodium	135–146 mmol/L
Urate	0.18–0.42 mmol/L (3.0–7.0 mg/dL)
Urea	2.5–6.7 mmol/L (8–25 mg/dL)

BLOOD GASES (ARTERIAL)

$P_a CO_2$	4.8–6.1 kPa (36–46 mmHg)
$P_a O_2$	10–13.3 kPa (75–100 mmHg)
[H^+]	35–45 nmol/L
pH	7.35–7.45
Bicarbonate	22–26 mmol/L

MEDICINE –
QUESTIONS

1. Rheumatology   3

2. Respiratory medicine   9

3. Endocrinology and diabetes   17

4. Renal medicine   27

5. Neurology   33

6. Haematology   45

7. Cardiovascular medicine   53

8. Gastroenterology and
    hepatobiliary medicine   61

Rheumatology

Single best answer

1. A 65-year-old man complains of pain and stiffness in his hands. On examination you note swelling of the distal interphalangeal joints and first carpometacarpal joint. What is the most likely diagnosis?

   A. Rheumatoid arthritis
   B. Osteoarthritis
   C. Psoriatic arthritis
   D. Gout
   E. Pseudogout

2. A 70-year-old woman presents with pain, swelling and stiffness in her knees. The latter is for a short period of time (< 30 minutes) worse early in the morning. Which investigation is most likely to lead to a diagnosis?

   A. Full blood count
   B. Erythrocyte sedimentation rate (ESR)
   C. Rheumatoid factor
   D. Knee X-ray
   E. C-reactive protein (CRP)

3. A 50-year-old man presents to his GP with pain in his hands. The GP notes small swellings on his distal and proximal interphalangeal joints. What is the next most appropriate step in management?

   A. Surgery
   B. Heat therapy
   C. Hydrotherapy
   D. Steroids
   E. Paracetamol

4. A 35-year-old woman presents with pain, swelling and stiffness in her hands. On examination you note swelling of the proximal interphalangeal joints as well as small nodules just below her elbows. Which investigation is most likely to lead to a diagnosis?

   A. Platelet count
   B. Haemoglobin levels
   C. Rheumatoid factor
   D. Antinuclear factor
   E. Erythrocyte sedimentation rate (ESR)

5. A 45-year-old woman presents to the GP with marked ulnar deviation of her hands. You note an obvious swan neck deformity of her fingers. What extra manifestation is she most likely to suffer from?

   A. Anaemia
   B. Pleural effusion
   C. Pericarditis
   D. Felty's syndrome
   E. Scleromalacia perforans

6. A 30-year-old man is diagnosed with rheumatoid arthritis. He mentions that the pain is difficult to cope with and has been ongoing for the last 4 months. What is the next most appropriate step in management?

   A. Non-steroidal anti-inflammatory drugs (NSAIDs)
   B. COX 2 inhibitors
   C. Surgery
   D. TNF-α blockers
   E. Methotrexate

7. A 23-year-old man presents with increasing pain, swelling and stiffness in his lower back. On examination you note a reduction in chest expansion and obvious kyphosis. What is the most likely diagnosis?

   A. Ankylosing spondylitis
   B. Psoriatic arthritis
   C. Osteoarthritis
   D. Reactive arthritis
   E. Enteropathic arthritis

8. A 20-year-old man returns from a trip to Amsterdam. He complains of pain in his knees as well as pain on passing urine. What is the most likely diagnosis?

   A. Ankylosing spondylitis
   B. Psoriatic arthritis
   C. Reactive arthritis
   D. Osteoarthritis
   E. Enteropathic arthritis

9. A 52-year-old man presents to his GP with pain in his hands. The GP notes swelling of his distal interphalangeal joints as well as pitting of his nails. What is the most likely diagnosis?

   A. Ankylosing spondylitis
   B. Psoriatic arthritis
   C. Osteoarthritis
   D. Reactive arthritis
   E. Enteropathic arthritis

10. A 30-year-old woman is admitted with a painful right knee. On examination the knee is warm to touch. Joint aspiration confirms the presence of a gram positive coccus. What is the most appropriate step in management?

    A. Non-steroidal anti-inflammatory drugs (NSAIDs)
    B. COX 2 inhibitors
    C. Bed rest
    D. Joint mobilization
    E. Flucloxacillin and fusidic acid

11. A 25-year-old woman presents with a rash on her nose and cheeks which she mentions gets worse in the sunlight. She also complains of joint pains in her hands. Which investigation is most likely to provide a diagnosis?

    A. Full blood count
    B. Antinuclear antibodies
    C. Anti-cardiolipin antibodies
    D. Complement levels
    E. Rheumatoid factor

12. A 45-year-old woman presents with pain in her hands. On examination you note thickening of her skin and tapering of her fingers. She also mentions that she has difficulty opening her mouth. Which investigation is most likely to support the diagnosis?

    A. Full blood count
    B. Hand X-ray
    C. Anti-centromere antibodies
    D. Anti-Jo 1 antibodies
    E. Anti-Ro antibodies

13. A 55-year-old man presents with weakness in his shoulders. He mentions he has difficulty raising his hands above his head. On examination you note a purple coloured rash on his face. What is the most likely diagnosis?

    A. Dermatomyositis
    B. Polmyositis
    C. Polymyalgia
    D. Overlap syndrome
    E. Systemic lupus erythematosus

14. A 60-year-old woman presents with weakness in her shoulders and lower limbs. She mentions she has difficulty walking upstairs and getting up from sitting. You suspect a diagnosis of polymyositis. Which investigation is most likely to confirm the diagnosis?

    A. Anti-Jo 1 antibodies
    B. Erythrocyte sedimentation rate (ESR)
    C. Electromyography (EMG)
    D. MRI spine
    E. Muscle biopsy

15. A middle aged woman presents with dry eyes and a dry mouth. She also mentions that her fingers feel colder than usual. Which antibody is usually present?

   A. Anti-Ro and Anti-La antibodies
   B. Anti-Jo 1 antibodies
   C. Anti-centrome antibodies
   D. Anti-cardiolipin antibodies
   E. Lupus anticoagulant

16. A child is taken to the GP by his mother. On examination the GP notes a rash on his legs and buttocks. The mother mentions he has difficulty walking and is particularly worried as she has noticed blood in his urine. The child was recently treated for a chest infection. What is the most likely diagnosis?

   A. Churg–Strauss syndrome
   B. Henoch–Schonlein purpura
   C. Microscopic polyangitis
   D. Polyarteritis nodosa
   E. Juvenile arthritis

17. A 55-year-old man presents with severe pain and swelling of his right big toe. He is obese and a heavy drinker. What is the most appropriate step in management?

   A. Allopurinol
   B. Probenecid
   C. Colchicine
   D. Non-steroidal anti-inflammatory drugs (NSAIDs)
   E. Steroids

18. An elderly woman who was diagnosed recently with haemochromatosis presents with pain and stiffness in her knees resembling osteoarthritis. Which of the following investigations is most likely to provide a diagnosis?

   A. White cell count
   B. Knee X-ray
   C. Serum calcium
   D. Joint fluid microscopy
   E. Uric acid levels

19. An Asian woman presents to the GP complaining of generalised muscle pains. She mentions she is struggling to walk and has difficulty rising from her chair. What is the most likely abnormality on serum investigation?

   A. High potassium
   B. High calcium
   C. Low sodium
   D. Low vitamin D
   E. Low magnesium

20. A 70-year-old woman has been diagnosed with osteoporosis. She is a heavy smoker and drinker. Her past history includes a fractured distal radius. What is the most appropriate step in management?

   A. Stop smoking
   B. Stop alcohol
   C. Hormone replacement therapy (HRT)
   D. Bisphosphonates
   E. Raloxifene

21. A 75-year-old man presents with significant pain in his legs. On examination you note bowing of his tibia. You suspect a diagnosis of Paget's disease. Which investigation is most likely to confirm your suspicion?

   A. Serum magnesium levels
   B. Serum alkaline phosphatase levels
   C. Vitamin B_{12} levels
   D. Serum folate levels
   E. Serum sodium levels

Extended matching questions

Theme: **Arthritis**

A. Enteropathic arthritis
B. Juvenile idiopathic arthritis
C. Tuberculous arthritis
D. Septic arthritis
E. Reactive arthritis
F. Osteoarthritis
G. Psoriatic arthritis
H. Rheumatoid arthritis
I. Gonococcal arthritis
J. *Salmonella* arthritis

For each scenario described below, choose the single most appropriate answer from the above list of options. Each option may be used once, more than once or not at all.

1. Involvement of the distal interphalangeal joints and first carpometacarpal joint of the hands. ☐

2. Involvement of the metacarpophalangeal joints and proximal interphalangeal joints of the hands. ☐

3. Involvement of the metacarpophalangeal joints and proximal interphalangeal joints of the hands with pitting of the nails. ☐

4. Involvement of the knee joint with visual discomfort and pain on passing urine. ☐

5. Involvement of the lower limb joints in a patient with ulcerative colitis. ☐

Theme: **Connective tissue disease**

A. Antiphospholipid syndrome
B. Systemic sclerosis
C. Systemic lupus erythematosus
D. Discoid lupus
E. Polymyositis
F. Dermatomyositis
G. Overlap syndrome
H. Sjögren's syndrome
I. Polymyalgia
J. Eczema

For each scenario described below, choose the single most appropriate answer from the above list of options. Each option may be used once, more than once or not at all.

1. A woman presenting with a butterfly rash and joint discomfort. ☐

2. A woman presenting with a red coloured facial rash made worse by sunlight. ☐

3. A 25-year-old woman with a history of three consecutive miscarriages. ☐

4. A 55-year-old man with a purple coloured rash around his eyes. ☐

5. A 65-year-old woman presenting with difficulty in opening her mouth and palpable swellings in her fingers. ☐

Theme: **Vasculitis**

A. Polymyalgia
B. Temporal arteritis
C. Kawasaki's disease
D. Wegener's granulomatosis
E. Churg–Strauss syndrome
F. Henoch–Schönlein purpura
G. Essential cryoglobulinaemia
H. Polyarteritis nodosa
I. Behçet's disease
J. Microscopic polyangiitis

For each scenario described below, choose the single most appropriate answer from the above list of options. Each option may be used once, more than once or not at all.

1. A 55-year-old man complaining of a history of stiffness and intense pain in his shoulder and back. ☐

2. A 55-year-old woman complaining of a sudden onset headache associated with a loss of pulsation in her temporal artery. ☐

3. A middle aged man with abdominal pain and deranged renal function. A renal biopsy confirms inflammation of medium sized arteries. ☐

4. A middle aged man presenting with generalised abdominal pain and haematuria. Urine dipstick reveals the presence of blood and protein.

An auto antibody screen reveals the presence of perinuclear antineutrophil cytoplasmic antibodies (pANCA). ☐

5. A 43-year-old woman presenting with mouth ulcers and red coloured painful lumps on her thighs. ☐

Theme: **Drugs**

A. Methotrexate
B. Penicillamine
C. Azathioprine
D. Sulfasalazine
E. Hydroxychloroquine
F. Auranofin
G. Sodium aurothiomalate
H. Diclofenac
I. Infliximab
J. Leflunomide

For each scenario described below, choose the single most appropriate answer from the above list of options. Each option may be used once, more than once or not at all.

1. Associated with mouth ulcers, proteinuria and thrombocytopenia. ☐

2. Associated with headaches and visual disturbances. ☐

3. A therapeutic agent associated with a blue-coloured skin discoloration in sunlight. ☐

4. Associated with male infertility and hepatitis. ☐

5. A therapeutic agent administered intramuscularly known to cause mouth ulcers and pulmonary fibrosis. ☐

Theme: **Back pain**

A. Prolapsed intervertebral disc
B. Spondylolisthesis
C. Spinal stenosis
D. Ankylosing spondylitis
E. Bacterial osteomyelitis
F. Myeloma
G. Cauda equina syndrome
H. Tuberculosis osteomyelitis
I. Osteoporosis
J. Paget's disease

For each scenario described below, choose the single most appropriate answer from the above list of options. Each option may be used once, more than once or not at all.

1. A middle aged woman presenting with low back pain, groin numbness and urinary retention. ☐

2. Associated with an aching pain in the lower back when walking with radiation into the lower limbs. The pain is eased by rest. ☐

3. A 23-year-old man presenting with sudden onset back pain after weight lifting which is exacerbated by movement and coughing. ☐

4. A 54-year-old man complaining of back stiffness and shooting pains down his legs which worsens throughout the day. On examination you note obvious lordosis and a waddling like gait. ☐

5. Pain and stiffness in the lower back known to affect late teens. ☐

Single best answer

1. A 65-year-old life-long smoker presents with a wheeze, breathlessness and sputum production. On examination you note reduced chest expansion bilaterally. He has lived in central London since the age of 10. Which of the following is most likely to be causing his symptoms?

   A. Living in the city
   B. Asthma
   C. Alpha 1 antitrypsin deficiency
   D. Chronic obstructive pulmonary disease (COPD)
   E. None of the above

2. A 60-year-old man with severe chronic obstructive pulmonary disease (COPD) is admitted with an acute exacerbation. What is the most appropriate initial investigation?

   A. CT chest scan
   B. Spirometry
   C. Arterial blood gas
   D. Peak flow
   E. Pulmonary function tests

3. A 68-year-old woman is admitted under your care with increasing breathlessness, wheeze and sputum production. She has chronic obstructive pulmonary disease (COPD). What is the next most appropriate step in management?

   A. 60% oxygen
   B. 24% oxygen
   C. Oral steroids
   D. Non-invasive positive-pressure ventilation
   E. Antibiotics

4. An overweight middle aged man presents to the GP after his wife complains about his loud snoring. He tends to drink large amounts of alcohol in the evenings before going to bed. Which of the following features is he most likely to complain of?

   A. Morning headaches
   B. Nocturnal choking
   C. Reduced libido
   D. Daytime sleepiness
   E. Personality changes

5. A child is admitted with a cough and sputum production which is thick, foul smelling and green in colour. The mother notes episodes of him coughing up blood. On examination he has notable finger clubbing with course crackles in both lung bases on auscultation. What is the most likely cause of his symptoms?

   A. Cystic fibrosis
   B. Inhaled foreign body
   C. Measles
   D. *Klebsiella*
   E. Whooping cough

6. You suspect bronchiectasis in a young patient. Which of the following investigations is most likely to confirm the diagnosis?

   A. Sputum culture
   B. Sweat test
   C. Bronchography
   D. Chest X-ray
   E. CT chest scan

7. A child recently diagnosed with cystic fibrosis is admitted following an exacerbation of his symptoms. What is the next most appropriate step in management?

   A. Prednisolone
   B. *N*-acetylcysteine
   C. Sodium re-absorption blockers
   D. Antibiotics
   E. Aminophylline

8. A teenager presents to the GP with symptoms indicative of cystic fibrosis. A sweat test is performed. Which of the following is diagnostic?

   A. A chloride value between 40 and 60 mmol/l
   B. A chloride value less than 40 mmol/l
   C. A sodium value of less than 60 mmol/l
   D. A sodium value above 60 mmol/l
   E. A sodium value between 40 and 60 mmol/l

9. A 35-year-old vet presents with a wheeze, cough and shortness of breath. He has smoked 10 cigarettes a day for 6 months. He likes to keep fit by running marathons. His grandfather had asthma as a child. He has lived in central London for the past year. Which of the following is the most likely cause of his condition?

   A. Family history
   B. Smoking
   C. Occupation
   D. Exercise
   E. City living

10. You suspect asthma in a 25-year-old woman. What is the most appropriate initial investigation to help confirm the diagnosis?

    A. Histamine provocation test
    B. Peak expiratory flow rate
    C. Spirometry
    D. Skin prick allergy test
    E. Chest X-ray

11. A known asthmatic presents to the GP complaining of gradually worsening of her symptoms. She is already taking a regular β_2 agonist inhaler. Her peak flow is 65% of her predicted value. What is the next most appropriate step in management?

    A. Long-acting β_2 agonist inhaler
    B. Low-dose inhaled steroid
    C. High-dose inhaled steroid
    D. Oral prednisolone
    E. Intravenous hydrocortisone

12. A woman is admitted to hospital with acute severe asthma. Her respiratory rate is greater than 25 breaths/min and peak flow is less than 50% of her predicted value. What is the next most appropriate step in management?

    A. Oral prednisolone
    B. Intravenous hydrocortisone
    C. Intravenous salbutamol
    D. Intravenous aminophylline
    E. Nebulised ipratropium

13. A middle aged woman is admitted to hospital with a cough, sputum production, fever and dyspnoea. A diagnosis of pneumonia is made. Which of the following organisms is most likely to account for her symptoms?

    A. *Streptococcus pneumoniae*
    B. *Haemophilus influenzae*
    C. *Legionella pneumophila*
    D. *Staphylococcus aureus*
    E. *Aspergillus fumigatus*

14. An elderly woman is admitted to hospital with pneumonia. The following are all risk factors used in predicting mortality in community acquired pneumonia EXCEPT?

    A. Urea greater than 7 mmol/l
    B. Age of 65 years
    C. Respiratory rate of 20 breaths per minute
    D. Blood pressure less than 90 systolic
    E. Confusion

15. A middle aged man presents with cough, sputum production, fever and dyspnoea. Red coloured papules are noted on the back of his hands. Routine blood investigations demonstrate that he is anaemic. Which of the following organisms is most likely to account for his condition?

    A. *Chlamydia pneumoniae*
    B. *Haemophilus influenzae*
    C. *Staphylococcus aureus*
    D. *Mycoplasma pneumoniae*
    E. *Legionella pneumophila*

16. A 42-year-old man presents to the GP with symptoms suggestive of pneumonia. He also complains of generalised muscular pains. He has many pets at home and mentions he recently bought two parrots. Which of the following organisms would account for his condition?

    A. *Chlamydia psittaci*
    B. *Haemophilus influenzae*
    C. *Staphylococcus aureus*
    D. *Mycoplasma pneumoniae*
    E. *Legionella pneumophila*

17. A 23-year-old known intravenous drug abuser is admitted with a fever, productive cough and dyspnoea. Which of the following organisms is most likely to account for his condition?

    A. *Chlamydia pneumoniae*
    B. *Haemophilus influenzae*
    C. *Staphylococcus aureus*
    D. *Mycoplasma pneumoniae*
    E. *Legionella pneumophila*

18. A 32-year-old man presents to the GP with a fever, productive cough and chest pain. He has recently been abroad to Dubai and stayed at a newly built hotel. He mentioned he had bouts of diarrhoea in the last few days of his trip which he put down to the foreign food. Which of the following organisms is most likely to account for his condition?

    A. *Chlamydia pneumoniae*
    B. *Haemophilus influenzae*
    C. *Staphylococcus aureus*
    D. *Mycoplasma pneumoniae*
    E. *Legionella pneumophila*

19. A 40-year-old man is diagnosed with a mild pneumonia. He has no known drug allergies. What is the most appropriate treatment?

    A. Amoxicillin
    B. Metronidazole
    C. Azithromycin
    D. Cefuroxime
    E. Flucloxacillin

20. You suspect pneumonia in a 35-year-old woman. Which of the following investigations is most likely to confirm the diagnosis?

    A. Blood culture
    B. Sputum culture
    C. White cell count
    D. Chest X-ray
    E. Arterial blood gas

21. An Asian man presents with a 2-month history of fever and a cough productive of blood tinged sputum. He has recently moved to the United Kingdom from abroad. What is the most likely causative organism?

    A. *Mycoplasma pneumoniae*
    B. *Streptococcus pneumoniae*
    C. *Mycobacterium avium intracellulare*
    D. *Mycobacterium tuberculosis*
    E. *Pneumocystis jiroveci*

22. A West Indian immigrant has recently been diagnosed with tuberculosis. Which of the following cells are solely responsible for engulfing bacilli and forming granulomatous lesions?

    A. Neutrophils
    B. Macrophages
    C. Langhans' giant cells
    D. Epithelioid cells
    E. T lymphocytes

11

23. An Asian immigrant presents with a fever and a cough productive of blood-tinged sputum. On examination you note an enlarged liver and enlarged cervical lymph nodes. A chest X-ray shows patchy shadowing in the upper zones. You suspect tuberculosis. What is the next most appropriate investigation you would order to confirm your suspicion?

    A. Bronchoscopy
    B. Sputum smear
    C. Mantoux test
    D. Lymph node biopsy
    E. CT chest scan

24. A middle aged man is diagnosed with tuberculosis. He has no known drug allergies. Which is the least likely drug to be included in the initial treatment?

    A. Ethambutol
    B. Pyrazinamide
    C. Streptomycin
    D. Rifampicin
    E. Isoniazid

25. A 55-year-old man has been recently diagnosed with tuberculosis. He has been started on quadruple therapy and complains of a colour change in his urine. What drug is most likely to be responsible for this?

    A. Rifampicin
    B. Isoniazid
    C. Ethambutol
    D. Pyrazinamide
    E. Streptomycin

26. An Afro Caribbean man presents with increasing dyspnoea. A chest X-ray shows bilateral hilar lymphadenopathy. Routine blood investigations demonstrate a raised serum calcium. Which of the following is also likely to be affected?

    A. Heart
    B. Central nervous system
    C. Bones and joints
    D. Liver
    E. Eyes

27. You suspect sarcoidosis in an Afro Caribbean man who presents with a cough and evidence of lymphadenopathy. Which of the following investigations is likely to be most useful in confirming a diagnosis?

    A. Abdominal X-ray
    B. Lung function tests
    C. Transbronchial biopsy
    D. Serum angiotensin converting enzyme (ACE)
    E. Lymph node biopsy

28. A middle aged man presents with exertional dyspnoea and a non-productive cough. On examination he has finger clubbing and fine inspiratory crackles are noted bi basally on auscultation. What is the most likely diagnosis?

    A. Asbestosis
    B. Pneumoconiosis
    C. Cryptogenic fibrosing alveolitis
    D. Extrinsic allergic alveolitis
    E. Sarcoidosis

29. Which of the following is the most common cause of extrinsic allergic alveolitis?

    A. Forking mouldy hay
    B. Handling pigeons
    C. Turning germinating barley
    D. Turning mushroom compost
    E. Contaminated humidifier systems in air conditioners

30. A ship-building-yard worker presents with breathlessness. A CT chest scan is ordered and a diagnosis of asbestos-induced lung damage is made. He is distraught with the diagnosis and wants to know if he is eligible for industrial injury benefits. Which of the following findings would allow him to pursue a claim?

    A. Pleural plaques
    B. Pleural effusion
    C. Asbestos bodies
    D. Bilateral diffuse pleural thickening
    E. None of the above

31. A 65-year-old woman presents with breathlessness and haemoptysis. She is diagnosed with squamous cell carcinoma of the lung. She has been a smoker for as long as she can remember. She has lived in central London for almost 30 years now and she worked in a ship-building yard for most of her working life. Both her father and mother died of lung cancer. Which of the following is the most likely cause of her cancer?

A. Smoking
B. Gender
C. Family history
D. Occupation
E. City living

32. A middle aged man is diagnosed with lung cancer. He worked in a ship-building yard for most of his life. He is distraught with the diagnosis as he says he has never smoked in his life. Which of the following types of lung cancer is he most likely to suffer from?

A. Squamous
B. Large cell
C. Adenocarcinoma
D. Alveolar cell
E. Small cell

33. A 53-year-old woman is diagnosed with lung cancer. Her main symptoms on presentation included breathlessness and haemoptysis. She complained of stretch marks on her abdomen and that her skin bruised easily. On examination you note purple abdominal striae. Which of the following types of lung cancer is she most likely to suffer from?

A. Squamous cell
B. Large cell
C. Adenocarcinoma
D. Alveolar cell
E. Small cell

34. A 63-year-old man is diagnosed with lung cancer. Which of the following extra pulmonary manifestations is he most likely to suffer from?

A. Clubbing
B. Dermatomyositis
C. Eaton–Lambert syndrome
D. Hypercalcaemia
E. Thrombophlebitis migrans

35. A 61-year-old man with a solitary lung nodule is referred for bronchoscopy. Biopsies from the mass reveal small cell lung cancer (SCLC). Staging investigations show localised disease with no spread to mediastinal nodes or involvement of either main bronchus or recurrent laryngeal nerve. What is the next most appropriate step in his management?

A. Surgery
B. Radiotherapy
C. Chemotherapy
D. Endoscopic laser therapy
E. Stenting

36. With regard to pleural fluid, which of the following is most important in determining whether an effusion is a transudate or exudate?

A. Bacterial count
B. Amylase levels
C. Malignant cells
D. Glucose levels
E. Protein levels

37. Which of the following typically causes a transudative pleural effusion?

A. Heart failure
B. Pneumonia
C. Bronchial carcinoma
D. Pancreatitis
E. Connective tissue disease

38. **A 45-year-old woman presents with shortness of breath and chest pain. She comments that she has recently travelled to Australia. An ECG demonstrates evidence of right heart strain. You suspect a pulmonary embolus. Which investigation is most likely to lead to a diagnosis?**

   A. CT pulmonary angiogram
   B. D dimers
   C. Ventilation perfusion scan
   D. Chest X-ray
   E. Arterial blood gas

Extended matching questions

Theme: **Pneumonia**

   A. *Mycoplasma pneumoniae*
   B. *Chlamydia psittaci*
   C. *Staphylococcus aureus*
   D. *Legionella pneumophila*
   E. *Haemophilus influenzae*
   F. Aspiration pneumonia
   G. *Pseudomonas aeruginosa*
   H. *Pneumocystis jiroveci*
   I. *Streptococcus pneumoniae*
   J. *Mycobacterium avium intracellulare*

For each scenario described below, choose the single most likely causative organism from the above list of options. Each option may be used once, more than once or not at all.

1. A 32-year-old man presenting with shortness of breath and feeling generally unwell. He has a known history of cystic fibrosis. ☐

2. A common cause of pneumonia in patients with chronic obstructive pulmonary disease (COPD). ☐

3. A middle aged man presenting with a cough and generalised muscular pains. He is known to be a keen collector of rare birds. ☐

4. An intravenous drug abuser presenting with shortness of breath and a fever. ☐

5. A middle aged woman having recently returned from Las Vegas presenting with a non-productive cough, fever and diarrhoea. ☐

Theme: **Drugs**

   A. Ethambutol
   B. Pyrazinamide
   C. Isoniazid
   D. Rifampicin
   E. Metronidazole
   F. Erythromycin
   G. Clarithromycin
   H. Flucloxacillin
   I. Tobramycin
   J. Ticarcillin

For each scenario described below, choose the single most likely drug from the above list of options. Each option may be used once, more than once or not at all.

1. Associated with induction of liver enzymes. ☐

2. Associated with blurred vision and colour blindness. ☐

3. An intravenous drug abuser diagnosed with pneumonia associated with patchy areas of consolidation on his chest X-ray. ☐

4. Known to cause liver inflammation and gout. ☐

5. A middle aged woman recently diagnosed with a stroke aspirates when given some water. ☐

Theme: **Lung cancer**

A. Eaton Lambert syndrome
B. Dermatomyositis
C. Herpes zoster
D. Acanthosis nigricans
E. Hypertrophic pulmonary osteoarthropathy
F. Horner's syndrome
G. Pancoast's tumour
H. Cushing's syndrome
I. Thrombophlebitis migrans
J. Clubbing

For each scenario described below, choose the single most appropriate answer from the above list of options. Each option may be used once, more than once or not at all.

1. A 75-year-old man recently diagnosed with lung cancer complaining of painful wrists and ankles. ☐

2. A middle aged man recently presenting with haemoptysis and shoulder pain. ☐

3. A 65-year-old woman presenting with breathlessness, haemoptysis and pigmented skin in her axillae. ☐

4. A middle aged woman with known lung cancer presenting with dropping of her upper eyelid, pupillary constriction and a sunken eye on the right side. ☐

5. A patient recently diagnosed with lung cancer presenting with lower limb weakness and difficulty in climbing stairs. ☐

Theme: **Diseases of the respiratory tract**

A. Bronchiectasis
B. Sinusitis
C. Rhinitis
D. Pharyngitis
E. Laryngotracheobronchitis
F. Influenza
G. Emphysema
H. Bronchitis
I. Asthma
J. Obstructive sleep apnoea

For each scenario described below, choose the single most appropriate answer from the above list of options. Each option may be used once, more than once or not at all.

1. Dilatation and destruction of lung tissue distal to terminal bronchioles. ☐

2. A 23-year-old man presenting with sudden onset cough, fever and muscular aches. ☐

3. Associated with a hoarse voice and barking cough. ☐

4. An 18-year-old woman with cystic fibrosis presenting with a cough productive of green coloured sputum. ☐

5. A middle aged man presenting with cough, chest tightness and wheeze. ☐

Theme: **Investigative findings**

A. Chronic obstructive pulmonary disease
B. Obstructive sleep apnoea
C. Sarcoidosis
D. Wegener's granulomatosis
E. Bronchiectasis
F. Cystic fibrosis
G. Extrinsic allergic alveolitis
H. Asthma
I. Cryptogenic fibrosing alveolitis
J. Pneumonia

For each scenario described below, choose the single most appropriate answer from the above list of options. Each option may be used once, more than once or not at all.

1. A middle aged woman with shortness of breath and a ground-glass appearance on her chest X-ray. ☐

2. A 55-year-old farmer presenting with a cough and shortness of breath. His chest X-ray demonstrates fluffy nodular shadowing. ☐

3. A life-long smoker with an FEV_1 to FVC ratio of 62% with an increase in FEV_1 of 12% following use of salbutamol. ☐

4. A 23-year-old woman presenting with a fever, cough and shortness of breath. Routine blood investigations reveal a white cell count of 23×10^9/l. A chest X-ray demonstrates evidence of patchy consolidation. ☐

5. A 45-year-old man presenting with haemoptysis. A chest X-ray reveals evidence of cavitation and routine blood investigations demonstrate increased levels of anti-neutrophil cytoplasmic antibodies. ☐

Endocrinology and diabetes

Single best answer

1. A middle aged man is diagnosed with a pituitary tumour following an MRI head scan. One of his complaints includes gradual loss of vision. With regard to his visual loss, which of the following features is he most likely to demonstrate?

   A. Paracentral scotoma
   B. Mononuclear field loss
   C. Bitemporal hemianopia
   D. Homonymous hemianopia
   E. Homonymous quadrantanopia

2. A 53-year-old woman is diagnosed with hypopituitarism. Which of the following hormones is most likely to be affected first?

   A. Follicle stimulating hormone (FSH) and luteinizing hormone (LH)
   B. Thyroid stimulating hormone (TSH)
   C. Adrenocorticotropic hormone (ACTH)
   D. Prolactin
   E. Growth hormone

3. A 65-year-old man is diagnosed with an under-active pituitary gland. Which of the following is the most common cause of hypopituitarism?

   A. Infection
   B. Vascular
   C. Immunological
   D. Trauma
   E. Neoplastic

4. A 25-year-old woman is diagnosed with hypopituitarism. Which of the following hormones is essential to replace first when managing her condition?

   A. Thyroid hormone
   B. Oestrogen
   C. Growth hormone
   D. Luteinizing hormone
   E. Follicle stimulating hormone

5. A 29-year-old man complains of headaches and visual disturbances. He also remarks that he can express milk from his breasts. What is the most appropriate initial investigation?

   A. MRI pituitary scan
   B. Visual field assessment by perimetry
   C. Thyroid function tests
   D. Serum prolactin level
   E. Serum testosterone level

6. A 42-year-old man complains of visual disturbances and headaches. He remarks his wedding ring feels tighter than usual. On examination you note a protruding jaw, interdental separation and spade like hands. Which investigation is most likely to confirm the diagnosis?

   A. Serum growth hormone
   B. Serum insulin like growth factor 1 (IGF 1)
   C. Serum prolactin
   D. Oral glucose tolerance test
   E. Visual field assessment by perimetry

7. A 40-year-old woman presents to her GP complaining of tiredness, weight gain and feeling unusually cold. On general examination the GP notes a slow relaxing ankle jerk. The GP diagnoses hypothyroidism. The patient enquires about the cause of her condition. Which of the following is the most likely cause of her hypothyroidism?

   A. Idiopathic
   B. Iodine deficiency
   C. Dyshormonogenesis
   D. Pituitary insufficiency
   E. Hashimoto's thyroiditis

8. A 35-year-old man complains of weight gain and feeling cold. Thyroid function tests demonstrate a low T4 and a raised thyroid stimulating hormone (TSH). He is also notably anaemic with a haemoglobin of 10.2 g/dl. What is the most likely type of anaemia he will demonstrate?

   A. Aplastic anaemia
   B. Macrocytic
   C. Microcytic
   D. Autoimmune haemolytic anaemia
   E. Non autoimmune haemolytic anaemia

9. A 55-year-old man with treated hypothyroidism presents with confusion. His hypothyroidism is due to an under active pituitary gland. Blood tests reveal a sodium of 128 mmol/l and a glucose of 2.8 mmol/l. Routine observations reveal a temperature of 35 °C. What is the most appropriate step in management?

   A. Sodium replacement
   B. Glucose replacement
   C. Intravenous T3 replacement
   D. Intravenous hydrocortisone
   E. Warmed intravenous fluids

10. A 35-year-old woman is diagnosed with an overactive thyroid gland. What is the most likely aetiological cause of her thyrotoxicosis?

    A. Toxic multinodular goitre
    B. Solitary toxic nodule
    C. De Quervain's thyroiditis
    D. Graves' disease
    E. Thyroiditis factitia

11. A 40-year-old woman complains of weight loss and heat intolerance. Routine blood investigations confirm a diagnosis of Graves' disease. Which of the following features are specific to this disease?

    A. Lid lag
    B. Tremor
    C. Proximal myopathy
    D. Atrial fibrillation
    E. Ophthalmoplegia

12. A 35-year-old man complains of weight loss and heat intolerance. On examination you note an obvious goitre and red coloured lesions on his shins. You suspect Graves' disease. Which investigation is most likely to lead to a diagnosis?

    A. Thyroid stimulating hormone (TSH)
    B. T4 and T3 levels
    C. Thyroid ultrasound
    D. Thyroid stimulating hormone receptor antibodies
    E. Thyroglobulin antibodies

13. A 32-year-old woman complains of weight loss and heat intolerance. She mentions her heart is always racing. A quick examination reveals marked exophthalmus. What is the next most appropriate step in management?

    A. Propanolol
    B. Carbimazole
    C. Radioactive iodine
    D. Surgery
    E. Propylthiouracil

14. A middle aged woman is diagnosed with hyperthyroidism. Her GP commences carbimazole. Which of the following is the most likely side effect of this medication?

    A. Rash
    B. Nausea and vomiting
    C. Arthralgia
    D. Jaundice
    E. Agranulocytosis

15. A 29-year-old woman is diagnosed with hyperthyroidism. She is currently 28 weeks pregnant. The following are all suitable treatments for hyperthyroidism EXCEPT?

    A. Carbimazole
    B. Propanolol
    C. Radioactive iodine
    D. Surgery
    E. Propylthiouracil

16. A 35-year-old woman has recently undergone radioactive iodine therapy for an overactive thyroid. Her condition deteriorates and she becomes notably restless and delirious. On examination she has a pulse rate of 120 beats/min and a temperature of 40 °C. She is severely dehydrated. What is the first most appropriate step in her management?

    A. Dexamethasone
    B. Potassium iodide
    C. Propranolol
    D. Carbimazole
    E. Intravenous fluids

17. A patient presents with exophthalmos and opthalmoplegia. She has a known history of hyperthyroidism. Which of the following is the first most appropriate step in management?

    A. Steroids
    B. Orbit irradiation
    C. Watchful waiting
    D. Lateral tarsorraphy
    E. Normalization of thyroid status

18. A 36-year-old woman presents with a significantly enlarged goitre. She complains of a discomfort in her neck as well as breathing difficulties. On examination you note a solitary nodule. She is worried about the possibility of cancer. Which of the following investigations is most likely to reveal such a diagnosis?

    A. Thyroid stimulating hormone (TSH)
    B. T4 and T3 levels
    C. Chest radiography
    D. Fine-needle aspiration for cytology
    E. Thyroid scan (^{125}I)

19. A 40-year-old woman presents with a goitre. On examination you note a nodule which feels hard and irregular in size. You also note the presence of enlarged cervical lymph nodes. Fine-needle aspiration confirms the presence of malignant cells. Routine blood investigations reveal a calcium level of 3.67 mmol/l. Which one of the following is the most likely type of her thyroid cancer?

    A. Papillary
    B. Follicular
    C. Anaplastic
    D. Medullary cell
    E. Lymphoma

20. A 35-year-old woman is diagnosed with thyroid cancer. Histological assessment confirms the diagnosis as anaplastic with pulmonary metastases. What is the next most appropriate step in management?

    A. Palliative
    B. Radioactive iodine
    C. Sub total thyroidectomy
    D. Total thyroidectomy
    E. Chemotherapy

21. A 43-year-old man is diagnosed with Cushing's syndrome. Which one of the following is most likely to be decreased or inhibited in this condition?

    A. Protein catabolism
    B. Free water clearance
    C. Circulating neutrophils
    D. Uric acid production
    E. Circulating lymphocytes

22. A 35-year-old woman complains of lethargy, low mood and loss of weight. On examination you note increased pigmentation of her buccal mucosa and skin creases. Her blood pressure drops to 85/60 mmHg from 122/63 mmHg on standing. Which of the following investigations is most likely to confirm her diagnosis?

    A. Serum urea and electrolytes
    B. Adrenal antibodies
    C. Abdominal X-ray
    D. Tetracosactide (synacthen) short test
    E. Tetracosactide (synacthen) long test

23. A middle aged man is diagnosed with adrenal gland insufficiency. What is the most likely aetiological cause for this condition?

    A. Autoimmune
    B. Adrenal gland tuberculosis
    C. Haemorrhage
    D. Pituitary disease
    E. Adrenal gland tumour

24. A middle aged woman is admitted to the medical admissions unit with severe abdominal pain and weakness. On examination she has a pulse rate of 120 beats/min, a blood pressure of 95/65 mmHg and a urine output of less than 30 ml/hour. Routine blood tests reveal a random plasma glucose of 3.0 mmol/l. You note deep pigmentation of her buccal mucosa and skin creases. Her GP referral letter comments that she has been feeling tired, low in mood and suffering weight loss for the past one month. What is the first most appropriate step in her management?

    A. Intramuscular hydrocortisone
    B. Intravenous glucose
    C. Intravenous hydrocortisone
    D. Intravenous dextrose
    E. Intravenous fludrocortisone

25. A 45-year-old gentleman is diagnosed with impaired adrenal function. He has been taking steroids on and off for the past 2 years for treatment of severe Crohn's disease. Which of the following investigations is most likely to reveal the cause of his adrenal failure?

    A. Urea and electrolytes
    B. Adrenal antibodies
    C. Abdominal X-ray
    D. Tetracosactide (synacthen) short test
    E. Tetracosactide (synacthen) long test

26. A 53-year-old woman complains that she has put on a considerable amount of weight over the past 2 months. She also mentions that her skin feels thin and bruises easily. On examination you note a plethoric complexion and purple striae on her abdomen. A 24-hour urinary cortisol is three times the upper limit of normal. What is the most likely cause of her condition?

    A. Adrenal adenoma
    B. Adrenal carcinoma
    C. Adrenal hyperplasia
    D. Pituitary adenoma
    E. Carcinoid tumour

27. A 45-year-old woman is diagnosed with Cushing's syndrome. Routine blood tests reveal a significantly raised adrenocorticotropic hormone (ACTH) level. High dose dexamethasone suppresses plasma cortisol after 48 hours. What is the most likely cause of her condition?

    A. Adrenal adenoma
    B. Adrenal carcinoma
    C. Adrenal hyperplasia
    D. Pituitary adenoma
    E. Carcinoid tumour

28. A 50-year-old man complains of feeling low in mood. On examination his blood pressure is 140/85 mmHg. His body mass index (BMI) is 31. He has purple streaks on his abdomen as well as pigmentation of skin creases. Investigations confirm Cushing's syndrome secondary to a pituitary adenoma. What is the next most appropriate step in management?

   A. External beam irradiation
   B. Aminoglutethimide
   C. Ketoconazole
   D. Metyrapone
   E. Surgical excision of tumour

29. A 30-year-old woman is admitted to accident and emergency complaining of nausea and headaches. She appears mildly confused and is unaware of her surroundings. On examination her blood pressure is 125/80 mmHg with no postural drop. Investigations show a serum sodium of 122 mmol/l, a low plasma osmolality, a urine osmolality which is much higher than plasma and a urinary sodium level which is greater than 30 mmol/l. What is the most likely cause of her symptoms?

   A. Renal tubular acidosis
   B. Glucocorticoid deficiency
   C. Syndrome of inappropriate ADH
   D. Renal failure
   E. Salt-wasting nephropathy

30. What is the most appropriate management of the patient described above?

   A. Furosemide
   B. Hypertonic saline
   C. Hypotonic saline
   D. Dimethylchlorotetracycline
   E. Fluid restriction

31. A 32-year-old man with a recent diagnosis of mania is treated with lithium. Three weeks later he returns complaining of feeling thirsty and going to pass urine up to 8 times a day. Which of the following investigations is most likely to confirm the diagnosis?

   A. Urine volume measurement
   B. Plasma sodium concentration
   C. Urine osmolality
   D. Plasma osmolality
   E. Water deprivation test

32. A 25-year-old woman complains of abdominal pain and non-specific bone pain for the past 2 weeks. She also mentions that she has been feeling generally low in herself. Routine blood tests reveal a raised parathyroid hormone level and a low vitamin D level. Her corrected serum calcium level is 2.01 mmol/l. What is the most likely diagnosis?

   A. Primary hyperparathyroidism
   B. Secondary hyperparathyroidism
   C. Tertiary hyperparathyroidism
   D. DiGeorge syndrome
   E. Pseudohypoparathyroidism

33. A 42-year-old woman with breast cancer complains of non-specific bone pain, abdominal discomfort and not opening her bowels for the past one week. Her GP decides to admit her. Upon arrival you note she is severely dehydrated and confused. Routine blood tests reveal a corrected serum calcium level of 4.0 mmol/l. What is the first most appropriate step in her management?

   A. Prednisolone
   B. Intravenous fluid replacement
   C. Bisphosphonates
   D. Calcitonin
   E. Phosphate

34. A 35-year-old man complains of numbness around his mouth. On examination you note opposition of his thumb, extension of his interphalangeal joints and flexion of his metacarpophalangeal joints. His corrected serum calcium is 1.70 mmol/l. What is the most likely cause of his symptoms?

    A. Osteomalacia
    B. Pseudohypoparathyroidism
    C. DiGeorge syndrome
    D. Idiopathic hypoparathyroidism
    E. Renal failure

35. You suspect primary hyperaldosteronism in a 65-year-old man with hypertension. Which of the following investigations is most important in helping to confirm such a diagnosis?

    A. Plasma aldosterone to renin ratio
    B. Plasma potassium
    C. Adrenal CT scan
    D. Adrenal MRI scan
    E. Urinary potassium

36. A 45-year-old man complains of headaches, sweating and nausea. On examination his pulse rate is 135 beats/min and his blood pressure is 138/95 mmHg. Routine blood tests reveal a random plasma glucose of 10.2 mmol/l. You suspect the possibility of a catecholamine producing tumour. Which of the following investigations is most likely to confirm the diagnosis?

    A. Clonidine suppression and glucagon stimulation test
    B. Abdominal CT scan
    C. Abdominal MRI scan
    D. 24-hour urinary collection of metanephrines
    E. Metaiodobenzylguanidine (mIBG) CT scintigraphy

37. A 57-year-old man presents to the GP complaining of feeling thirsty, weight loss and passing urine up to nine times a day. His body mass index (BMI) is 32. Routine blood tests reveal a random blood glucose of 12.2 mmol/l. What is the next most appropriate step in management?

    A. Diet therapy
    B. Glibenclamide
    C. Insulin
    D. Acarbose
    E. Rosiglitazone

38. A 55-year-old man has been recently diagnosed with type II diabetes. His body mass index (BMI) is 35.5. What is the most appropriate medical management?

    A. Glibenclamide
    B. Metformin
    C. Acarbose
    D. Repaglinide
    E. Pioglitazone

39. A newly diagnosed diabetic is commenced on metformin. What is the most common side effect of this drug?

    A. Lactic acidosis
    B. Hypoglycaemic
    C. Flatulence
    D. Bloating
    E. Diarrhoea

40. A 22-year-old man complains of feeling tired, thirsty and going to pass urine more frequently than normal. His fasting plasma glucose is 14.2 mmol/l. What is the next most appropriate step in management?

    A. Acarbose
    B. Rapid-acting insulin
    C. Diet alone
    D. Intermediate-acting insulin
    E. Oral hypoglycaemics

41. A diabetic patient on insulin is found unconscious at home. He is immediately transferred to hospital. Routine blood tests reveal a glucose level of 1.9 mmol/l. What is the next most appropriate step in management?

    A. Intramuscular glucagon
    B. Oral carbohydrate
    C. Intravenous dextrose
    D. Diazoxide
    E. Octreotide

42. A 32-year-old diabetic man on insulin is admitted to hospital having been found unconscious at home. He quickly regains consciousness on arrival. On examination his eyes are sunken and his tongue appears dry. His breathing is deep at a rate of 25 breaths/min. His blood pressure is 110/65 mmHg. Routine blood tests reveal a plasma glucose of 22 mmol/l. You perform an arterial blood gas which demonstrates a pH of 7.10, a PCO_2 of 3.5 kPa and a bicarbonate of 19 mmol/l. What is the next most appropriate step in his management?

    A. Intravenous saline
    B. Intravenous insulin
    C. Sodium bicarbonate infusion
    D. Intravenous colloids
    E. Intramuscular glucagon

43. A 65-year-old diabetic man who is a poor clinic attendee presents to his GP complaining of blurred vision. Fundoscopy reveals the presence of yellow coloured exudates as well as cotton wool spots. What is the most likely diagnosis?

    A. Background retinopathy
    B. Maculopathy
    C. Pre-proliferative retinopathy
    D. Proliferative retinopathy
    E. Cataracts

44. A 55-year-old diabetic woman complains of numbness, tingling and pain in her toes and hands. She comments that it is particularly worse at night. Examination reveals bilateral loss of sensation on the palms and soles. What is the most likely diagnosis?

    A. Autonomic neuropathy
    B. Acute painful neuropathy
    C. Diabetic mononeuropathy
    D. Diabetic amyotrophy
    E. Symmetrical sensory neuropathy

45. A 29-year-old diabetic woman is trying for a baby. She visits her GP to ask about whether her diabetes may affect her pregnancy. Diabetes may result in the following complications during pregnancy EXCEPT?

    A. Macrosomia
    B. Hydramnios
    C. Respiratory distress syndrome
    D. Pre-eclampsia
    E. Neonatal hyperglycaemia

46. A 31-year-old man complains of sweating and palpitations. He remarks he often sees double. Routine blood tests reveal a fasting plasma glucose of 2.2 mmol/l. He undergoes an abdominal CT scan which reveals the presence of a pancreatic tumour. What is the next most appropriate step in management?

    A. Surgical excision of tumour
    B. Diazoxide
    C. Octreotide
    D. Chemotherapy
    E. Radiotherapy

Extended matching questions

Theme: **Pituitary disease**

A. Pituitary apoplexy
B. Sheehan's syndrome
C. Empty sella syndrome
D. Kallmann's syndrome
E. Pituitary tumour
F. Syphilis
G. Haemochromatosis
H. Sarcoidosis
I. Lymphocytic hypophysitis
J. Anorexia

For each scenario described below, choose the single most appropriate answer from the above list of options. Each option may be used once, more than once or not at all.

1. Associated with loss of smell and colour blindness. ☐

2. Associated with severe blood loss following childbirth. ☐

3. A middle aged woman presenting with sudden onset headaches, nausea and visual disturbances. ☐

4. A 37-year-old obese woman with known hypertension presenting with sudden onset headaches. A head MRI scan reveals an unusually small pituitary gland. ☐

5. A middle aged man presenting with enlarged hands and feet. On further questioning he complains of visual disturbances and headaches. ☐

Theme: **Thyroid disease**

A. Hashimoto's thyroiditis
B. Lymphocytic thyroiditis
C. Dyshormonogenesis
D. Myxoedema coma
E. Graves' disease
F. Plummer's disease
G. de Quervain's thyroiditis
H. Thyroid cancer
I. Thyroid crisis
J. Toxic multinodular goitre

For each scenario described below, choose the single most appropriate answer from the above list of options. Each option may be used once, more than once or not at all.

1. Over activity of the thyroid gland associated with fever and neck pain. ☐

2. A common cause of hyperthyroidism associated with IgG antibodies. ☐

3. A common cause of hypothyroidism associated with auto antibody formation and goitre formation. ☐

4. A middle aged woman presenting with enlargement of the thyroid gland and a markedly raised serum calcium. ☐

5. A woman with known hyperthyroidism presenting with fever, tachycardia and restlessness following radioactive iodine therapy. ☐

Theme: **Diabetic complications**

A. Background retinopathy
B. Maculopathy
C. Pre proliferative retinopathy
D. Proliferative retinopathy
E. Symmetrical sensory neuropathy
F. Autonomic neuropathy
G. Acute painful neuropathy
H. Diabetic mononeuropathy
I. Diabetic amyotrophy
J. Mononeuritis multiplex

For each scenario described below, choose the single most appropriate answer from the above list of options. Each option may be used once, more than once or not at all.

1. A common form of neuropathy affecting the toes and soles of the feet. ☐

2. Associated with cotton wool spots and venous beading. ☐

3. Associated with blot haemorrhages and yellow coloured exudates. ☐

4. A diabetic patient complaining of wasting of his quadriceps muscles. ☐

5. A diabetic patient presenting with a burning sensation in his anterior lower limbs which is generally worse at night. ☐

Theme: **Drugs**

A. Glibenclamide
B. Tolbutamide
C. Metformin
D. Acarbose
E. Rosiglitazone
F. Repaglinide
G. Protamine insulin
H. Insulin lispro
I. Insulin aspart
J. Pioglitazone

For each scenario described below, choose the single most appropriate answer from the above list of options. Each option may be used once, more than once or not at all.

1. Associated with diarrhoea and abdominal bloating. This agent may also result in elevated serum transaminase levels. ☐

2. Associated with diarrhoea and lactic acidosis. ☐

3. First line agent in the treatment of type II diabetes in obese individuals. ☐

4. A drug which works via closure of K$^+$ ATP channels but is best avoided in elderly people. ☐

5. An insulin releasing agent developed from glibenclamide. ☐

Theme: **Investigations**

A. Thyroid function tests
B. Oral glucose tolerance test
C. Plasma aldosterone levels
D. Serum urea and electrolytes
E. Short synacthen test
F. Long synacthen test
G. Dexamethasone suppression test
H. Urine and plasma osmolality
I. Fasting blood glucose
J. 24 hour urinary collection of metanephrines

For each scenario described below, choose the single most appropriate answer from the above list of options which would help in making a diagnosis. Each option may be used once, more than once or not at all.

1. A middle aged man presenting with enlargement of his hands and feet. ☐

2. A 34-year-old obese gentleman presenting with a plethoric complexion and purple coloured striae on his abdomen. ☐

3. Associated with sudden onset headaches, palpitations and sweating. ☐

4. A middle aged woman presenting with weight loss and lethargy. Examination reveals hyper-pigmentation of oral mucosa and skin creases. ☐

5. A 45-year-old man presenting with increased urinary frequency and thirst. Blood glucose levels are normal. ☐

Single best answer

1. A 45-year-old man complains of breathlessness and feeling tired for the past one week. He also remarks that he has not been passing as much urine as usual. On clinical examination he is not dehydrated. He has a serum creatinine of 500 μmol/l. Urine analysis reveals a urine osmolality of 650 mOsm/kg and a urine sodium of 15 mmol/l. You diagnose acute renal failure. What is the least likely cause of his renal failure?

   A. Decreased cardiac output
   B. Severe liver failure
   C. Hypovolaemia
   D. Renal artery obstruction
   E. Acute tubular necrosis

2. A middle aged woman presents with breathlessness for the last one week. She also comments that she has been feeling more tired than usual and that she has been passing urine infrequently. On examination you note that her skin is pale and pigmented with several small bruises. What is the most appropriate initial investigation?

   A. Urea and electrolytes
   B. Urine Stix testing and microscopy
   C. Serum calcium, phosphate and uric acid
   D. Full blood count
   E. Renal ultrasound

3. A 51-year-old man is diagnosed with acute renal failure. He has recently been suffering from diarrhoea and vomiting and has lost his appetite. He takes captopril for his high blood pressure. He is oliguric with a urine output of less than 300 ml/day. Routine blood tests reveal a potassium of 6.5 mmol/l. What is the first most appropriate step in his management?

   A. Treat his high potassium
   B. Fluid replacement
   C. Diuretics
   D. Withdraw captopril
   E. Nutrition replacement

4. A patient with acute renal failure is referred for dialysis. The following are all indications for dialysis EXCEPT?

   A. Severe metabolic acidosis
   B. Uncontrollable hyperkalaemia
   C. Pulmonary oedema
   D. Pericarditis
   E. Anaemia

5. A 56-year-old man is diagnosed with acute renal failure. The cause of this was attributed to interstitial nephritis. The following drugs all cause interstitial nephritis EXCEPT?

   A. NSAIDs
   B. ACE inhibitors
   C. Allopurinol
   D. Penicillin
   E. Cimetidine

6. A 65-year-old man complains of waking up in the night to pass urine for the past 3 weeks. He feels generally quite tired and complains of muscle weakness. Routine blood tests reveal a serum calcium of 1.76 mmol/l, a serum phosphate of 3.4 mmol/l, a low vitamin D level and a raised parathyroid hormone level. You diagnose renal osteodystrophy. Which of the following radiological signs is least likely?

   A. 'Rugger jersey' spine
   B. Subperiosteal erosions

27

C. 'Pepperpot' skull

D. Brown tumours

E. Pseudofractures

7. A 57-year-old woman is diagnosed with chronic renal failure. Which of the following is most likely to suggest a chronic picture?

A. Bruising

B. Skin pigmentation

C. Pericarditis

D. Confusion

E. Low serum calcium

8. A 67-year-old diabetic patient complains of bone and muscle pain for the last 4 weeks. She remarks that she feels more tired than usual and is constantly itching. Routine blood investigations reveal a serum creatinine of 255 mmol/l and a haemoglobin of 8.7 g/dl. In addition, her vitamin D level is low. What is the most appropriate step in her management?

A. Review of diabetic medication

B. Reduction of protein intake

C. Erythropoietin injections

D. Referral for dialysis

E. Vitamin D analogues

9. A 68-year-old man with chronic renal failure is referred for peritoneal dialysis. What is the most likely complication of this form of dialysis?

A. Cardiovascular disease

B. Peritonitis

C. Amyloidosis

D. Shoulder pain

E. Carpal tunnel syndrome

10. A 51-year-old man complains of pain in his loins and passing blood in his urine for the past 2 weeks. There is a strong family history of polycystic kidney disease (PKD). On examination his blood pressure is recorded as 160/95 mmHg. What investigation is most likely to confirm the diagnosis of PKD?

A. 24 hour ambulatory blood pressure monitoring

B. Urea and electrolytes

C. Urine Stix testing and microscopy

D. Renal ultrasound

E. Excretion urography

11. A 67-year-old man complains of loin pain and passing blood in his urine for the past 1 week. On examination you note the presence of large irregular kidneys. You are concerned about the possibility of polycystic kidney disease. What is the usual mode of inheritance of this condition?

A. Autosomal recessive

B. X-linked recessive

C. Autosomal dominant

D. X-linked dominant

E. Y-linked

12. A 57-year-old man presents with haematuria, loin pain and a solid mass in his right flank. Excretion urography demonstrates the presence of a space occupying lesion. What is the most appropriate step in her management?

A. Medroxyprogesterone acetate

B. Surgery

C. Interleukin 2

D. Alpha interferon

E. Radiotherapy

13. A 70-year-old man complains of waking up in the night to pass urine, non specific bone pain and weight loss. He mentions that there is often a delay in initiating urination and a sense of incomplete voiding. What is the most appropriate initial investigation after a digital rectal examination?

A. Urea and electrolytes

B. Serum prostate specific antigen (PSA)

C. Renal ultrasound

D. Transrectal ultrasound

E. Excretion urography

14. An 85-year-old man complains of waking up in the night to pass urine. He mentions that there is often a delay in initiating urination and a sense of incomplete evacuation. On examination you note the presence of a hard

irregular prostate. An examination under anaesthesia is performed which confirms prostate cancer. Subsequent staging reveals the tumour has extended through the capsule with involvement of the seminal vesicles. What is the most appropriate step in his management?

A. Goserelin
B. Cyproterone acetate
C. Orchidectomy
D. External beam radiotherapy
E. Surgery

15. A 30-year-old man complains of a painful swelling in his right testicle. Routine blood tests reveal a Beta HCG level which is higher than normal. Surgical exploration and subsequent histological examination of the testis reveals the presence of cystic spaces. What is the most likely diagnosis?

A. Seminoma
B. Teratoma
C. Sertoli cell adenoma
D. Leydig cell adenoma
E. Testicular torsion

16. A 31-year-old man complains of a painless swelling in his left testicle. Routine blood tests reveal a Beta HCG level which is higher than normal. In addition his alpha fetoprotein level is markedly raised. What is the most likely diagnosis?

A. Seminoma
B. Teratoma
C. Sertoli cell adenoma
D. Leydig cell adenoma
E. Testicular torsion

17. A 29-year-old man presents with a painless swelling in his left testicle. He complains of a cough and shortness of breath. Ultrasound scanning reveals the presence of a testicular tumour. Surgical exploration and subsequent histological examination reveals no cystic spaces. In addition to an orchidectomy what is the next most appropriate step in management?

A. Chemotherapy
B. Radiotherapy

C. Watchful waiting
D. Goserelin
E. Cyproterone acetate

18. A 35-year-old woman complains of accidentally passing urine when she coughs or laughs. She also mentions that she often has a strong desire to pass urine and finds it difficult to hold it. She has given birth to three children. Urine Stix testing reveals a trace of protein. What is the most likely diagnosis?

A. Genuine stress incontinence
B. Urge incontinence
C. Stress incontinence
D. Overflow incontinence
E. Urinary tract infection

19. A 61-year-old man complains of hesitancy, a poor stream and terminal dribbling when passing urine. On examination you note the presence of a distended bladder palpable suprapubically. Which investigation is most likely to lead to a diagnosis?

A. Radionuclide studies
B. Cystometrogram
C. Abdominal ultrasound
D. Uretography
E. Cystoscopy

20. A 43-year-old man with gout complains of severe intermittent loin pain and microscopic haematuria which has lasted for several hours. What is the initial most appropriate step in management?

A. Fluid replacement
B. Allopurinol
C. Pain relief
D. Shock wave lithotripsy
E. Nephrolithotomy

21. A 23-year-old marathon runner complains of severe intermittent loin pain and vomiting soon after a training session for her next marathon. On examination she is severely dehydrated.

Which of the following investigations is most likely to lead to a diagnosis?

A. Serum calcium levels

B. Abdominal X-ray of kidneys, ureters and bladder (KUB)

C. Urea and electrolytes

D. Mid-stream specimen of urine (MSU) for culture and sensitivity

E. 24-hour urine collection for calcium

22. A 24-year-old woman complains of urinary frequency and dysuria. What organism is the most likely cause of her symptoms?

A. *Escherichia coli*

B. *Proteus mirabilis*

C. *Klebsiella aerogenes*

D. Enterococci

E. *Staphylococcus saprophyticus*

23. A 30-year-old man complains of urinary frequency, dysuria and suprapubic tenderness for the past one week. What is the most appropriate initial investigation?

A. Urine microscopy and culture

B. Excretion urography

C. Abdominal X-ray

D. Micturating cystourethrography

E. Cystoscopy

24. An elderly man is catheterised having failed to pass urine for the past 2 days. Soon after he becomes significantly confused and complains of generalised loin pain. On examination he is pyrexial with a temperature of 39.5°C. What is the most appropriate step in his management?

A. High fluid intake

B. Trimethoprim

C. Nitrofurantoin

D. Amoxicillin

E. Gentamicin

25. A 4-year-old boy presents with swelling of his ankles, genitals and abdomen. On examination you also note slight swelling of his arms. His jugular venous pressure (JVP) is not raised. His mother mentions that his urine appears frothy. Which investigation is most likely to lead to a diagnosis?

A. 24-hour urinary protein and serum albumin measurement

B. Urine microscopy

C. Plasma lipids measurement

D. Urea and electrolytes

E. Renal ultrasound

26. A 6-year-old boy is diagnosed with nephrotic syndrome. What is the most likely cause of this condition?

A. Amyloidosis

B. Penicillamine

C. Glomerulonephritis

D. Diabetes

E. Systemic lupus erythematosus

27. A 60-year-old man with rheumatoid arthritis presents with generalised swelling of his ankles and abdomen. You request a urine sample which shows a raised protein level but no evidence of infection. Routine blood tests reveal a serum albumin of 22 g/l. What is the first most appropriate step in management?

A. Sodium restricted diet

B. Ciclosporin

C. High-protein diet

D. Albumin infusion

E. Cyclophosphamide

28. A 60-year-old man complains of haematuria. On examination his blood pressure is recorded as 190/110 mmHg. Urine microscopy reveals the presence of red cell casts. What is the next most appropriate step in management?

A. Corticosteroids

B. Immunosuppressives

C. Blood pressure control

D. Dietary protein restriction

E. Referral for dialysis

Extended matching questions

Theme: **Renal disease**

A. Acute nephritic syndrome
B. Nephrotic syndrome
C. Urinary tract infection
D. Tubulointerstitial nephritis
E. Renal stone disease
F. Urinary tract obstruction
G. Polycystic kidney disease
H. Medullary sponge kidney
I. Renal carcinoma
J. Renal hypertension

For each scenario described below, choose the single most appropriate answer from the above list of options. Each option may be used once, more than once or not at all.

1. An uncommon condition associated with dilatation of the collecting ducts in the papillae and cyst formation. ☐

2. An autosomal dominant condition associated with cyst formation and mutations in the PKD1 gene. ☐

3. A 7-year-old boy presenting with haematuria and proteinuria following a sore throat. ☐

4. A condition associated with proteinuria, oedema and hypoalbuminaemia. ☐

5. A middle aged man presenting with polyuria and nocturia. He is known to suffer from rheumatoid arthritis for which he takes non-steroid anti-inflammatory drugs (NSAIDs). ☐

Theme: **Complications of renal failure**

A. Anaemia
B. Osteomalacia
C. Osteoporosis
D. Osteosclerosis
E. Amyloidosis
F. Autonomic neuropathy
G. Cardiomyopathy
H. Peptic ulceration
I. Acute pancreatitis
J. Gout

For each scenario described below, choose the single most appropriate answer from the above list of options. Each option may be used once, more than once or not at all.

1. Associated with an increase in trabeculae typically in cancellous bone. ☐

2. Associated with the deposition of insoluble fibrillar protein deposition and diagnosed by Congo Red staining of tissues. ☐

3. A multifactorial pathogenesis associated with depressed bone marrow activity and decreased erythropoietin formation. ☐

4. A 65-year-old man with known renal failure presenting with postural hypotension, nausea and vomiting. ☐

5. A condition characterized by incomplete mineralization of osteoid tissue. ☐

Theme: **Clinical features of renal disease**

A. Acute nephritic syndrome
B. Nephrotic syndrome
C. Acute renal failure
D. Tubulointerstitial nephritis
E. Renal stone disease
F. Urinary tract obstruction
G. Chronic renal failure
H. Medullary sponge kidney
I. Renal carcinoma
J. Renal hypertension

For each scenario described below, choose the single most appropriate answer from the above list of options. Each option may be used once, more than once or not at all.

1. Typical features include swelling of the ankles, genitals and abdomen. ☐

2. Associated with shortness of breath, generalised lethargy and bone pain. ☐

3. Typical features include haematuria, loin pain and a mass in the flank. ☐

4. May be associated with pain and swelling of the big toe. ☐

5. Typical features include haematuria, proteinuria and oedema in children following a sore throat. ☐

Theme: Investigations

A. Urea and electrolytes
B. Prostate-specific antigen
C. Urine microscopy and culture
D. Magnetic resonance angiography
E. X-ray of the kidneys, ureters and bladder
F. Renal ultrasound
G. Renal biopsy
H. Serum albumin
I. Cystoscopy
J. Urodynamics

For each scenario described below, choose the single most appropriate answer from the above list of options. Each option may be used once, more than once or not at all.

1. A patient with known ischaemic heart disease taking ACE inhibitors who subsequently develops renal failure. ☐

2. A 24-year-old long-distance runner presenting with severe right-sided groin pain and vomiting. ☐

3. A 65-year-old man presenting with a poor urinary stream, terminal dribbling and hesitancy. ☐

4. A 75-year-old woman presenting with confusion, pain on passing urine and fever. ☐

5. A 35-year-old woman presenting with urinary incontinence following coughing or standing. ☐

Theme: Management of renal disease

A. Haemodialysis
B. Peritoneal dialysis
C. Surgery
D. Alpha blockers
E. Amoxicillin
F. Analgesia
G. Prednisolone
H. Haemofiltration
I. Transplantation
J. Antihypertensives

For each scenario described below, choose the single most appropriate answer from the above list of options. Each option may be used once, more than once or not at all.

1. A 60-year-old gentleman presenting with frequency, nocturia and post-void dribbling. ☐

2. A 22-year-old marathon runner presenting with severe left-sided loin pain. ☐

3. An elderly gentleman presenting with fever, confusion and dysuria. ☐

4. A condition associated with proteinuria and hypoalbuminaemia. ☐

5. The mainstay form of treatment in individuals presenting with haematuria, loin pain and a mass in the flank. ☐

Single best answer

1. A 35-year-old woman complains of generalised facial weakness along with difficulties in chewing. On examination you note ptosis and a slow downward drift of her outstretched arms. In addition you observe that her speech appears slower than normal. What is the most appropriate initial investigation?

   A. Acetylcholine receptor antibodies
   B. Electromyography (EMG)
   C. Muscle biopsy
   D. Creatine kinase levels
   E. Head CT scan

2. A 45-year-old lawyer complains of difficulty in releasing his grasp after shaking peoples' hands. What term most appropriately describes this?

   A. Myositis
   B. Muscular dystrophy
   C. Myaesthenia
   D. Myopathy
   E. Myotonia

3. A 7-year-old boy presents with difficulty in running and in rising to an erect position from the floor. His mother mentions that to become upright he often uses his hands to climb up his legs. What is the most likely diagnosis?

   A. Limb girdle dystrophy
   B. Facioscapulohumeral dystrophy
   C. Duchenne muscular dystrophy
   D. Becker muscular dystrophy
   E. Myotonia congenita

4. A 32-year-old alcoholic complains of numbness and tingling sensation in his hands. On general examination you note nystagmus. What is the most likely diagnosis?

   A. Vitamin B6 deficiency
   B. Vitamin B1 deficiency
   C. Vitamin B12 deficiency
   D. Vitamin A deficiency
   E. Vitamin C deficiency

5. A 45-year-old man presents with a one week history of progressive weakness and numbness in his distal limbs. On examination you note areflexia and muscle weakness but with normal sensation. Nerve conduction studies demonstrate slowing of motor conduction with segmental demyelination. You decide to perform a lumbar puncture. What is the most likely finding on cerebrospinal fluid (CSF) analysis?

   A. Normal protein, normal glucose, normal cell count
   B. Low protein, raised glucose, raised cell count
   C. Low protein, low glucose, low cell count
   D. Raised protein, normal glucose, raised cell count
   E. Raised protein, normal glucose, normal cell count

6. A 54-year-old woman with diabetes presents with pain and tingling in her right hand. On examination you note wasting of her thenar muscles. Which nerve is most likely to be affected?

   A. Radial
   B. Ulnar
   C. Median
   D. Brachial
   E. Musculocutaneous

7. A 65-year-old man presents with weakness in his hands and arms. On examination you note significant wasting and fasciculation. You suspect the possibility of motor neurone disease. Which investigation is most likely to lead to a diagnosis?

   A. Electromyography (EMG)
   B. Muscle biopsy
   C. Creatine kinase levels
   D. Head CT scan
   E. None of the above

8. A 32-year-old man presents with ataxia, dysarthria and visual disturbance. On examination you note absent lower limb tendon reflexes and an up going plantar response. You also note absence of joint position and vibration sense in his lower limbs. A visual examination demonstrates nystagmus and pale coloured optic discs. What is the most likely diagnosis?

   A. Cauda equina lesion
   B. Friedrich's ataxia
   C. Syringomyelia
   D. Syringobulbia
   E. Spinal cord compression

9. A 40-year-old woman presents with difficulty in walking. Neurological examination reveals significant weakness in her legs as well as notable spasticity. In addition you note a loss of sensation to pain and temperature in her upper limbs. Which investigation is most likely to lead to a diagnosis?

   A. Spinal MRI scan
   B. Spinal X-ray
   C. Spinal CT scan
   D. Muscle biopsy
   E. Electromyography (EMG)

10. A middle aged woman presents with back pain and weakness in her legs. On examination you note a loss of sensation below the level of L1. She complains that she finds it difficult to control her bladder and on occasions accidentally passes urine. What is the most likely cause for her symptoms?

    A. Epidural abscess
    B. Paget's disease
    C. Myeloma
    D. Glioma
    E. Neurofibroma

11. A 54-year-old woman presents with back pain and weakness in her legs. On examination you note significant spasticity in her legs. Appropriate imaging demonstrates the presence of a vertebral lesion. What is the most appropriate step in management?

    A. Dexamethasone
    B. Surgical decompression
    C. Physiotherapy
    D. Neck brace
    E. Baclofen

12. A 38-year-old man complains of headaches that typically last for 4 weeks followed by a period of remission. He describes the headache as being quite severe and located primarily around his right eye. During such episodes he suffers from watering of his eye as well as significant redness. What is the most likely diagnosis?

    A. Trigeminal neuralgia
    B. Giant-cell arteritis
    C. Cluster headache
    D. Migraine
    E. Tension headache

13. A 65-year-old woman complains of a headache and scalp tenderness when she combs her hair. She also suffers from jaw pain while eating and has noticed that her vision is intermittently poor. What is the most likely diagnosis?

    A. Trigeminal neuralgia
    B. Giant-cell arteritis
    C. Cluster headache
    D. Migraine
    E. Tension headache

14. A 60-year-old woman complains of a headache and scalp tenderness when she combs her hair. On examination you note her temporal arteries are tender, firm and pulseless. What is the next most appropriate step in management?

   A. Paracetamol
   B. Triptans
   C. Ergotamine
   D. Pizotifen
   E. Steroids

15. A 61-year-old woman complains of a headache and scalp tenderness when she combs her hair. She presents as an emergency due to sudden loss of vision in her right eye. Routine blood investigations reveal an erythrocyte sedimentation rate (ESR) of 65 mm/h. You perform a routine fundoscopy assessment. What is most likely to be seen on fundoscopy?

   A. Cherry-red spot
   B. Flame-shaped haemorrhages
   C. Cotton wool spots
   D. Silver wiring
   E. Papilloedema

16. A 28-year-old woman complains of a throbbing headache accompanied by nausea, vomiting and difficulty looking at bright lights. Prior to her headache she recalls seeing flashes and jagged lines. What is the most likely diagnosis?

   A. Trigeminal neuralgia
   B. Giant-cell arteritis
   C. Cluster headache
   D. Migraine
   E. Tension headache

17. A 30-year-old man complains of a throbbing headache and visual loss. He mentions that the headache comes on after eating chocolate biscuits which he is very fond of. What is the most likely aetiological cause for his headache?

   A. Serotonin
   B. Adrenaline
   C. Noradrenaline
   D. Dopamine
   E. Acetylcholine

18. A 35-year-old man complains of a 2-day history of headaches. During the consultation he begins to experience a headache which he describes as throbbing in nature. He also mentions he feels nauseous and his vision is deteriorating. His past medical history includes ischaemic heart disease. What is the next most appropriate step in management?

   A. Sumatriptan
   B. Ergotamine
   C. Methysergide
   D. Paracetamol and metoclopramide
   E. Pizotifen

19. A 63-year-old man accompanied by his wife presents with headaches and vomiting. His wife is keen to mention that he has become generally slow and that his personality is not what it used to be. She is worried as he is beginning to show little interest in his usual hobbies. He is referred for a CT head scan which reveals the presence of a tumour. What is the most likely site of his tumour?

   A. Temporal lobe
   B. Parietal lobe
   C. Frontal lobe
   D. Occipital lobe
   E. Cerebellum

20. A 55-year-old man presents with headache, vomiting and papilloedema. He describes the headache as getting worse when he coughs but decreasing when he stands up. A CT head scan reveals the presence of a tumour. What additional findings may there be on neurological examination?

   A. II nerve palsy
   B. III nerve palsy
   C. IV nerve palsy
   D. V nerve palsy
   E. VII nerve palsy

21. A 65-year-old woman complains of a sudden onset severe headache and an intolerance of bright lights. On examination you note neck stiffness. Routine observations reveal a temperature of 38.5°C. You suspect meningitis. What is the most likely organism responsible for her symptoms?

    A. *Neisseria meningitidis*
    B. *Staphylococcus aureus*
    C. *Streptococcus pneumoniae*
    D. *Listeria monocytogenes*
    E. Enterovirus

22. A 10-year-old boy presents with a headache and difficulty when looking at bright lights. On examination you note neck stiffness and a non blanching rash on his abdomen. He is pyrexial with a temperature of 39°C. There is no known history of drug allergies. What is the next most appropriate step in management?

    A. Paracetamol
    B. Cefotaxime
    C. Ampicillin
    D. Benzylpenicillin
    E. Chloramphenicol

23. A 19-year-old university student complains of a headache and a stiff neck. He also mentions he finds it difficult to look at bright lights. Observations reveal a temperature of 39°C. What is the most appropriate initial investigation?

    A. Blood culture
    B. Lumbar puncture
    C. Viral serology
    D. Head CT scan
    E. Syphilis serology

24. A 23-year-old university student is diagnosed with meningitis of bacterial aetiology. The cause has been assigned as bacterial. What is the most likely finding on cerebrospinal fluid (CSF) analysis?

    A. Lymphocytes, increased protein, normal glucose
    B. Lymphocytes, decreased protein, increased glucose
    C. Lymphocytes, normal protein, normal glucose
    D. Polymorphs, normal protein, normal glucose
    E. Polymorphs, increased protein, decreased glucose

25. A 35-year-old man presents with blurred vision and right sided eye pain. In addition he mentions he experiences a 'pins and needles'-like sensation on occasions. The following are all sites which may be affected in his condition EXCEPT?

    A. Optic nerve
    B. Periventricular white matter
    C. Spinal cord
    D. Cerebellum
    E. Peripheral nerves

26. A 32-year-old man presents with blurred vision and right-sided eye pain. In addition he complains of numbness and weakness in his legs. What is the most appropriate initial investigation?

    A. MRI brain scan
    B. Electrophysiology
    C. Lumbar puncture
    D. CT brain scan
    E. Cerebral angiography

27. A 31-year-old woman is diagnosed with multiple sclerosis following investigations which include a lumbar puncture. What is the most likely finding on cerebrospinal (CSF) analysis?

    A. Decreased polymorphs
    B. Monoclonal bands
    C. Increased glucose
    D. Decreased protein
    E. Oligoclonal bands

28. A 32-year-old man complains of a tremor when he holds a glass or spoon. He notices it improves when he drinks alcohol. What is the most likely diagnosis?

   A. Chorea
   B. Hemiballismus
   C. Myoclonus
   D. Benign essential tremor
   E. Tic

29. A 45-year-old man with Parkinson's disease complains of a jerky movement which spreads from one part of his body to the other ever since he was started on treatment for his condition. What is the most likely diagnosis?

   A. Chorea
   B. Hemiballismus
   C. Myoclonus
   D. Benign essential tremor
   E. Tic

30. A 35-year-old woman with epilepsy was witnessed as having a sudden jerking movement of her right arm while she fell asleep. What is the most likely diagnosis?

   A. Chorea
   B. Hemiballismus
   C. Myoclonus
   D. Benign essential tremor
   E. Tic

31. A 30-year-old man complains of prolonged spasms of muscle contraction. He is now receiving botulinum toxin which has improved his symptoms dramatically. What is the most likely diagnosis?

   A. Chorea
   B. Hemiballismus
   C. Myoclonus
   D. Dystonia
   E. Tic

32. A 65-year-old woman presents with a hand tremor. She has slowed considerably in day to day activities and now requires support for activities of daily living. On examination you note an expressionless face, slowness of movements and marked rigidity in her upper limbs. What is the initial most appropriate step in management?

   A. Bromocriptine
   B. Selegiline
   C. Amantadine
   D. Benzhexol
   E. Levodopa

33. A 62-year-old man presents with a shuffling gait and reduced arm swing. On examination you note a resting tremor. Which neurotransmitter is he most likely to be lacking?

   A. Dopamine
   B. Serotonin
   C. Noradrenaline
   D. Adrenaline
   E. Acetylcholine

34. A 53-year-old schizophrenic presents with a resting hand tremor. On examination you note slowness of movements, marked rigidity in his upper limbs and an inability to move his eyes vertically. What is the most likely diagnosis?

   A. Drug-induced parkinsonism
   B. Idiopathic parkinsonism
   C. Parkinsonism plus
   D. Methylphenyltetrahydropyridine (MPTP)-induced parkinsonism
   E. Postencephalitic parkinsonism

35. A 28-year-old man presents to accident and emergency following a fitting episode. His girlfriend witnessed the event and described it as a jerking action of his entire body. She mentioned the event did not last long. After the episode the gentleman remembers feeling drowsy and that his tongue was sore. What is the most likely diagnosis?

   A. Tonic clonic seizure
   B. Absence seizure
   C. Simple partial seizure

D. Complex partial seizure

E. Myoclonic seizure

36. A 7-year-old girl was witnessed by her father as having episodes where she suddenly stopped what she was doing, stared and then regained normal activity. What is the most likely diagnosis?

    A. Tonic clonic seizure

    B. Absence seizure

    C. Simple partial seizure

    D. Complex partial seizure

    E. Myoclonic seizure

37. A 45-year-old man presents following a fitting episode. He described it as a jerking like movement which began in his right hand and spread to the left side of his body. Following the episode he mentioned his upper limbs felt weak. What is the most likely diagnosis?

    A. Tonic clonic seizure

    B. Absence seizure

    C. Focal motor seizure

    D. Complex partial seizure

    E. Myoclonic seizure

38. A 39-year-old woman presents following a fitting episode. She recalls experiencing the smell of burning rubber during the event. What is the most likely diagnosis?

    A. Tonic clonic seizure

    B. Absence seizure

    C. Simple partial seizure

    D. Complex partial seizure

    E. Myoclonic seizure

39. A 32-year-old man is diagnosed with grand mal epilepsy. He is started on appropriate treatment. After 4 weeks he complains of hair loss. Routine blood investigations reveal an alanine aminotransferase (ALT) of 55 U/l, an aspartate aminotransferase (AST) of 55 U/l, an alkaline phosphatase (ALP) of 140 U/l and a

bilirubin of 3 mg/dl. Which drug is most likely to be responsible for these findings?

    A. Phenytoin

    B. Carbamazepine

    C. Ethosuximide

    D. Sodium valproate

    E. Vigabatrin

40. A 36-year-old man is diagnosed with grand mal epilepsy. He is started on appropriate treatment. During a routine review with his GP, blood investigations reveal a folate of 1.8 µg/l and a low vitamin D level. Which drug is most likely to be responsible for these findings?

    A. Phenytoin

    B. Carbamazepine

    C. Ethosuximide

    D. Sodium valproate

    E. Vigabatrin

41. A 34-year-old man is diagnosed with epilepsy. He is started on appropriate treatment. He goes to see his GP complaining of a generalised skin rash and 'night terrors'. Which drug is most likely to be responsible for this?

    A. Phenytoin

    B. Carbamazepine

    C. Ethosuximide

    D. Sodium valproate

    E. Vigabatrin

42. A known epileptic is admitted to accident and emergency following two consecutive seizures. Since the episode he has failed to regain consciousness. He has a history of poor compliance with medication. As the house officer on call you attempt to obtain intravenous access but fail. What is the next most appropriate step in management?

    A. Phenytoin

    B. Enobarbital

    C. Clonazepam

    D. Lorazepam

    E. Diazepam

43. A known epileptic is admitted to accident and emergency following two consecutive seizures. Since the episode he has failed to regain consciousness. He is known to drink heavily. What is the most appropriate initial investigation?

A. Serum electrolytes
B. Head CT scan
C. Lumbar puncture
D. Blood glucose
E. Blood cultures

44. A 55-year-old man presents with a sudden onset severe headache. On examination you note neck stiffness and that his right eye is abducted and looking down. Fundoscopy assessment reveals papilloedema. What is the most appropriate initial investigation?

A. Head CT scan
B. Head MRI scan
C. Lumbar puncture
D. Cerebral angiography
E. Visual field assessment by perimetry

45. A 54-year-old man presents with a sudden onset severe headache. On examination you note neck stiffness. A lumbar puncture is performed which reveals a yellow coloured supernatant after centrifugation of the CSF. What is the most likely diagnosis?

A. Intracerebral haemorrhage
B. Subarachnoid haemorrhage
C. Subdural haematoma
D. Extradural haematoma
E. None of the above

46. A 38-year-old alcoholic presents following a serious fall. He complains of a severe headache. On examination he appears drowsy and confused. What is the most likely diagnosis?

A. Intracerebral haemorrhage
B. Subarachnoid haemorrhage
C. Subdural haematoma
D. Extradural haematoma
E. None of the above

47. A 35-year-old man was found unconscious following a boxing match. He regains consciousness while in accident and emergency. During neurological assessment he rapidly deteriorates and becomes less aware of his surroundings. Which artery is most likely to have been ruptured?

A. Anterior cerebral
B. Middle cerebral
C. Posterior cerebral
D. Vertebral
E. Middle meningeal

48. A 62-year-old man presents with weakness on his right side. His symptoms however dramatically improve within 24 hours. What is the most likely diagnosis?

A. Stroke
B. Stroke in evolution
C. Minor stroke
D. Transient ischaemic attack
E. Completed stroke

49. A 60-year-old woman is diagnosed as having had a transient ischaemic attack arising from emboli in her internal carotid artery. She is likely to display all of the following features EXCEPT?

A. Amaurosis fugax
B. Aphasia
C. Hemiparesis
D. Hemisensory loss
E. Transient global amnesia

50. A 45-year-old obese man presents with right sided weakness, loss of sensation and visual disturbances. On examination you note increased tone, brisk reflexes and an up going plantar response. Which artery is most likely to be occluded?

A. Anterior cerebral
B. Middle cerebral
C. Posterior cerebral
D. Vertebral
E. Middle meningeal

51. A 53-year-old man presents with sudden onset vomiting and vertigo. On examination you note left-sided facial numbness and a diminished gag reflex. There is also reduced sensitivity to pain and temperature on the right side and evidence of a broad-based ataxic gait. Which artery is most likely to be occluded?

    A. Anterior cerebral
    B. Middle cerebral
    C. Posterior cerebral
    D. Posterior inferior cerebellar artery
    E. Middle meningeal

52. A diabetic life-long smoker presents with weakness on his right side. On examination you note an audible bruit in his internal carotid artery. What is the most appropriate initial investigation?

    A. Head CT scan
    B. Plasma glucose
    C. Carotid Doppler
    D. Urea and electrolytes
    E. Magnetic resonance angiography

53. An obese life-long smoker presents with a 12-hour history of right-sided weakness, loss of sensation and visual disturbances. On examination you note increased tone, brisk reflexes and an up-going plantar response. His blood pressure is 145/95 mmHg. A head CT scan reveals the presence of a cerebral infarct. What is the next most appropriate step in management?

    A. Antihypertensives
    B. Thrombolysis
    C. Heparin
    D. Warfarin
    E. Aspirin

54. A 32-year-old alcoholic presents to accident and emergency. On examination his speech is notably confused. His eyes open spontaneously and he withdraws to pain. What is his Glasgow Coma Scale Score?

    A. 9
    B. 10
    C. 11

D. 12
E. 13

55. A 35-year-old man presents with visual disturbance. He is later diagnosed with multiple sclerosis. What is the most likely type of his visual loss?

    A. Scotoma
    B. Bitemporal hemianopia
    C. Homonymous hemianopia
    D. Homonymous quadrantanopia
    E. None of the above

56. A 45-year-old man presents with visual disturbance. A CT head scan reveals a temporal lobe lesion. What is the most likely type of his visual loss?

    A. Scotoma
    B. Bitemporal hemianopia
    C. Homonymous hemianopia
    D. Homonymous quadrantanopia
    E. None of the above

57. A 32-year-old man is found unconscious at his home. He is immediately transferred to accident and emergency. On examination he is noted to have bilateral pupillary constriction. The following are all causes of pupil constriction EXCEPT?

    A. III nerve palsy
    B. Horner's syndrome
    C. Argyll Robertson pupil
    D. Opiate addiction
    E. Lesion at the pons

58. A 31-year-old woman presents with ptosis of her right eye. On examination you note that her right eye is abducted, pointing down and fixed to light. Which artery is most likely to be affected in this presentation?

    A. Anterior cerebral
    B. Middle cerebral
    C. Posterior cerebral
    D. Posterior communicating
    E. Middle meningeal

59. A 56-year-old woman presents with left-sided facial weakness. On examination you note dribbling from the corner of her mouth and that she is unable to close her eyes. She complains of hearing disturbance and you observe the presence of vesicles in her left ear. What is the most likely diagnosis?

A. Otitis media
B. Bell's palsy
C. Ramsay Hunt syndrome
D. Guillain–Barré syndrome
E. Otitis externa

60. A middle aged man complains of a sensation whereby his surroundings are revolving around him. He was recently prescribed gentamicin following a severe episode of pneumonia. What structure is most likely to be affected in his condition?

A. Labyrinth
B. VIII cranial nerve
C. Brainstem
D. Cerebellum
E. Basal ganglia

61. A middle aged man is diagnosed with a pseudobulbar palsy. The following are all findings of such a condition EXCEPT?

A. Dysarthria
B. Dysphagia
C. Nasal regurgitation
D. Exaggerated jaw jerk
E. Tongue fasciculations

62. A middle aged man with multiple sclerosis presents with an ataxic broad based gait. He is likely to demonstrate the following signs EXCEPT?

A. Intention tremor
B. Vertical nystagmus
C. Dysarthria
D. Pendular reflexes
E. Decreased tone

Extended matching questions

Theme: Cranial nerve lesions

A. I
B. II
C. III
D. IV
E. V
F. VI
G. VII
H. VIII
I. IX
J. X

For each scenario described below, choose the single most appropriate answer from the above list of options. Each option may be used once, more than once or not at all.

1. Associated with unilateral ptosis and a 'down and out' pupil. ☐

2. Known to cause loss of taste on the anterior two thirds of the tongue. ☐

3. Associated with diplopia when looking down and away from the affected side. ☐

4. Associated with unilateral visual loss in the form of an area of depressed vision within the visual field. ☐

5. Associated with unilateral sensory loss on the face and tongue. ☐

Theme: Diseases of the peripheral nerves

A. Vitamin B_6 deficiency
B. Vitamin B_1 deficiency
C. Vitamin B_{12} deficiency
D. Charcot Marie Tooth disease
E. Guillain–Barré syndrome

F. Carpal tunnel syndrome

G. Mononeuritis multiplex

H. Amyloidosis

I. HIV associated neuropathy

J. Autonomic neuropathy

For each scenario described below, choose the single most appropriate answer from the above list of options. Each option may be used once, more than once or not at all.

1. A diabetic patient presenting with pain and numbness in her hands, in addition to wasting of her thenar muscles. ☐

2. Associated with distal limb wasting and weakness. In advanced cases, the legs may resemble inverted champagne bottles. ☐

3. Associated with weakness and complaints of numbness in the distal limbs. Additional features include respiratory muscle weakness and postural hypotension. ☐

4. Seen commonly in individuals with a long standing history of alcohol abuse. ☐

5. A sensory neuropathy seen occasionally in individuals on isoniazid therapy. ☐

Theme: **Diseases of the muscle**

A. Limb girdle dystrophy

B. Facioscapulohumeral dystrophy

C. Myasthenia gravis

D. Dystrophia myotonica

E. Myotonia congenita

F. Cushing's syndrome

G. Hypothyroidism

H. Hyperthyroidism

I. Osteomalacia

J. Duchenne muscular dystrophy

For each scenario described below, choose the single most appropriate answer from the above list of options. Each option may be used once, more than once or not at all.

1. Presents in early childhood with weakness in the proximal leg muscles. ☐

2. Fatigability of proximal limb muscles in association with IgG acetylcholine receptor antibodies. ☐

3. An autosomal dominant condition characterized by distal muscle weakness and myotonia. ☐

4. An autosomal dominant condition characterized by myotonia in childhood. ☐

5. An autosomal recessive disorder associated with abnormal muscle function of the shoulder and pelvic girdle. ☐

Theme: **Epilepsy**

A. Grand mal

B. Petit mal

C. Myoclonic seizure

D. Jacksonian motor seizure

E. Temporal lobe epilepsy

F. Status epilepticus

G. West syndrome

H. Juvenile myoclonic epilepsy

I. Frontal lobe epilepsy

J. Lennox Gastaut syndrome

For each scenario described below, choose the single most appropriate answer from the above list of options. Each option may be used once, more than once or not at all.

1. A patient presenting with muscle jerking and incontinence of urine. ☐

2. Commonly seen in childhood whereby the individual ceases activity and stares for a few seconds. ☐

3. Associated with jerking movements beginning in the corner of the mouth and spreading to involve the limbs on the opposite side. ☐

4. Phenytoin is the first line treatment in this form of epilepsy. ☐

5. Associated with feelings of unreality or undue familiarity. ☐

Theme: **Extrapyramidal diseases**

A. Idiopathic Parkinson's disease

B. Multiple sclerosis

C. Drug-induced Parkinson's disease

D. Parkinsonism plus

E. Benign essential tremor

F. Chorea

G. Huntington's disease

H. Hemiballismus

I. Myoclonus

J. Tics

For each scenario described below, choose the single most appropriate answer from the above list of options. Each option may be used once, more than once or not at all.

1. A condition associated with signs of parkinsonism and an inability to move the eyes vertically or laterally. ☐

2. Associated with violent swinging movement of one side of the body. ☐

3. An autosomal dominant condition associated with a defective gene on chromosome 4. ☐

4. Brief repeated stereotypical movements involving the face and shoulders. ☐

5. A condition typically presenting in adult life associated with perivenular plaques of demyelination. ☐

36. A two-year-old boy of Middle Eastern origin is referred to the paediatric outpatient department by his GP following an abnormal blood count. The GP mentions that there is a strong family history of thalassaemia. On examination you note evidence of an enlarged maxilla and prominent frontal bones. What is the most likely diagnosis?

   A. Alpha thalassaemia
   B. Beta thalassaemia minor
   C. Beta thalassaemia intermedia
   D. Beta thalassaemia major
   E. Sickle cell disease

37. A 19-year-old girl with known sickle cell disease presents to the accident and emergency department with severe bone and chest pain following a viral infection. On examination you note she is mildly dehydrated. Her blood pressure and pulse are stable and oxygen saturation is 99% on room air. What is the next most appropriate step in management?

   A. Fluid replacement
   B. Analgesia
   C. Oxygen
   D. Antibiotics
   E. Aspirin

38. A 34-year-old woman with systemic lupus erythematosus is found to be anaemic. Which investigation is most likely to lead to a diagnosis?

   A. Coombs' test
   B. Serum ferritin level
   C. Blood film
   D. Vitamin B12 level
   E. Serum folate level

39. A patient with newly diagnosed autoimmune haemolytic anaemia is started on treatment. The haematologist notes that the patient's autoantibodies attach to red blood cells at a temperature of 29°C. Which management plan would you instigate first?

   A. Steroids
   B. Splenectomy
   C. Azathioprine
   D. Avoidance of cold exposure
   E. Cyclophosphamide

40. A 42-year-old man is diagnosed with warm antibody autoimmune haemolytic anaemia. Which of the following antibodies are components of this form of anaemia?

   A. IgG
   B. IgA
   C. IgM
   D. IgD
   E. IgE

Extended matching questions

Theme: Anaemia

A. Iron deficiency
B. Vitamin B12 deficiency
C. Aplastic anaemia
D. Paroxysmal nocturnal haemoglobinuria
E. Autoimmune haemolytic anaemia
F. Glucose-6-phosphate dehydrogenase deficiency
G. Sickle cell disease
H. Thalassaemia
I. Hereditary spherocytosis
J. Hereditary elliptocytosis

For each scenario described below, choose the single most appropriate answer from the above list of options. Each option may be used once, more than once or not at all.

1. Associated with a pancytopenia and a hypocellular bone marrow. ☐

2. An autosomal dominant condition associated with increased red cell osmotic fragility. ☐

3. Associated with jaundice and splenomegaly. The blood film may demonstrate the presence of cigar shaped blood cells. ☐

4. An X-linked disorder associated with neonatal jaundice and haemolysis due to ingestion of fava beans. ☐

5. A type of anaemia which occurs due to deficiency of CD59 and delay accelerating factor proteins. ☐

Theme: **Lymphadenopathy**

A. Epstein–Barr virus
B. Cytomegalovirus
C. Lymphoma
D. Leukaemia
E. Tuberculosis
F. HIV virus
G. Toxoplasmosis
H. Sarcoidosis
I. Carcinoma
J. Rheumatoid arthritis

For each scenario described below, choose the single most appropriate answer from the above list of options. Each option may be used once, more than once or not at all.

1. A disease of young adults associated with a sore throat, headache and a macular rash. ☐

2. A viral infection associated with depletion of CD4 helper lymphocytes. ☐

3. Characterised by malignant B and T lymphocytes with symptoms of anaemia, infection and bleeding. ☐

4. Associated with neoplastic cell formation in the bone marrow as result of a variety of genetic and environmental factors. ☐

5. A form of herpes virus that may result in fever, lethargy, diarrhoea and vomiting. ☐

Theme: **Splenomegaly**

A. Schistosomiasis
B. Leukaemia
C. Myelofibrosis
D. Malaria
E. Tuberculosis
F. Rheumatoid arthritis
G. Gaucher's disease
H. Kala azar
I. Endocarditis
J. Typhoid

For each scenario described below, choose the single most appropriate answer from the above list of options. Each option may be used once, more than once or not at all.

1. A disease associated with snail vectors which release cercariae that penetrate the skin to cause a papular rash. ☐

2. A condition prevalent in Asia and associated with dry wart-like hyper-pigmented skin lesions. ☐

3. A disease widespread in the tropics associated with red blood cell rupture by sporozoites. ☐

4. A lipid storage disease known to cause thrombocytopenia, bone pain and neurodegenerative effects. ☐

5. A middle aged woman presenting with abdominal pain, diarrhoea and confusion. On examination you note the presence of rose spots on the trunk. ☐

Single best answer

1. A 73-year-old woman complains of sudden onset chest pain. On examination you note her pulse is regular at 53 beats/min. You request an ECG which demonstrates a time interval of 3 seconds between each consecutive P wave. What is the most likely diagnosis?

   A. Sick sinus syndrome
   B. First degree AV block
   C. Mobitz type 1 block
   D. Mobitz type 2 block
   E. Complete heart block

2. A 63-year-old man complains of gradual onset chest pain. On examination you note his pulse is regular at 60 beats/min. You request an ECG which demonstrates an increasing PR interval which eventually culminates in an absent QRS complex after the P wave. What is the most likely diagnosis?

   A. Sick sinus syndrome
   B. First degree AV block
   C. Mobitz type 1 block
   D. Mobitz type 2 block
   E. Complete heart block

3. A 57-year-old man comes to his GP concerned about his general health. He is particularly worried as there is a strong family history of heart disease. The GP performs an ECG which shows a prolonged PR interval of 0.3 seconds. What is the most likely diagnosis?

   A. Sick sinus syndrome
   B. First degree AV block
   C. Mobitz type 1 block
   D. Mobitz type 2 block
   E. Complete heart block

4. You are a house officer on call when a nurse bleeps you to review an ECG. The ECG demonstrates an intermittent absence of the QRS complex but no evidence of progressive PR interval increase. What is the most likely diagnosis?

   A. Sick sinus syndrome
   B. First degree AV block
   C. Mobitz type 1 block
   D. Mobitz type 2 block
   E. Complete heart block

5. You are a house officer on call when you are bleeped to see a patient complaining of dizziness. On further questioning the patient comments that he has blacked out on several occasions in the past. You perform an ECG which shows regular P and QRS complexes occurring independently of one another. What is the most likely diagnosis?

   A. Sick sinus syndrome
   B. First degree AV block
   C. Mobitz type 1 block
   D. Mobitz type 2 block
   E. Complete heart block

6. You are a medical student attending a teaching session on ECG interpretation. The consultant tells you that a patient was admitted to the coronary care unit with an atrial rate of 300 beats/min and ventricular rate of 150 beats/min. What is the most likely diagnosis?

   A. Atrial flutter
   B. First degree AV block
   C. Mobitz type 1 block
   D. Mobitz type 2 block
   E. Complete heart block

7. You are a house officer on call when you are asked to review a patient in the coronary care unit. You note that the patient has an atrial rate of 300 beats/min and a ventricular rate of 150 beats/min. The nurse says this is of new onset. Which management plan would you instigate first?

   A. Sotalol
   B. Radiofrequency catheter ablation
   C. Procainamide
   D. Lignocaine
   E. Electrical cardioversion

8. A 57-year-old Bangladeshi patient is admitted to accident and emergency with palpitations. He speaks very little English but tells you he has a 'heart problem'. On examination you note his pulse is irregular at 145 beats/min. An ECG is performed which demonstrates no P waves. Which management plan would you instigate first?

   A. Bisoprolol
   B. Flecainide
   C. Radiofrequency catheter ablation
   D. Procainamide
   E. Lignocaine

9. A 37-year-old woman is complaining of palpitations following recent surgery. On examination her pulse rate is regular at 175 beats/min and blood pressure is stable at 125/70 mmHg. She tells you she was seen the night before by the on call cardiologist for the same problem. Her past medical history includes asthma. You request an ECG which shows normal shaped QRS complexes but no P waves. What is the next most appropriate step in management?

   A. Adenosine
   B. Verapamil
   C. Carotid sinus massage
   D. DC cardioversion
   E. Flecainide

10. While on call you are bleeped to see a patient who has had a massive bleed PR. On examination you note he is drowsy with a blood pressure of 65/40 mmHg and pulse rate of 130 beats/min. While you obtain intravenous access he arrests. The nurse calls the crash team and you commence CPR. After 2 minutes you note QRS complexes on the cardiac monitor but no evidence of a pulse. What is the next most appropriate step in management?

    A. Administration of colloid
    B. DC Shock 200 J
    C. Amiodarone 300 mg IV
    D. Adrenaline 1 mg IV
    E. Atropine 1 mg IV

11. A 42-year-old man presents with shortness of breath and haemoptysis. On examination you note a loud first heart sound and a rumbling mid diastolic murmur at the apex. What is the most likely diagnosis?

    A. Mitral stenosis
    B. Mitral regurgitation
    C. Aortic stenosis
    D. Aortic regurgitation
    E. Tricuspid stenosis

12. A 55-year-old woman presents with shortness of breath on exertion and fatigue. On examination you note a soft first heart sound and a pansystolic murmur at the apex radiating to her axilla. What is the most likely diagnosis?

    A. Mitral stenosis
    B. Mitral regurgitation
    C. Aortic stenosis
    D. Aortic regurgitation
    E. Tricuspid stenosis

13. A 62-year-old man presents with angina and dyspnoea. On examination you note an ejection systolic murmur at the upper right sternal border radiating to his neck. What is the most likely diagnosis?

    A. Mitral stenosis
    B. Mitral regurgitation
    C. Aortic stenosis
    D. Aortic regurgitation
    E. Tricuspid stenosis

14. A 55-year-old woman presents with dyspnoea and orthopnoea. On examination you note a blowing early diastolic murmur at the left sternal edge. What is the most likely diagnosis?

   A. Mitral stenosis
   B. Mitral regurgitation
   C. Aortic stenosis
   D. Aortic regurgitation
   E. Tricuspid stenosis

15. A 42-year-old man is reviewed in the outpatient cardiology department following a recent echocardiogram (echo). The echo demonstrates right ventricular dysfunction. On examination you note an elevated JVP in addition to a pansystolic murmur at the lower left sternal edge. What is the most likely diagnosis?

   A. Mitral stenosis
   B. Mitral regurgitation
   C. Tricuspid regurgitation
   D. Aortic stenosis
   E. Aortic regurgitation

16. A 62-year-old man presents with angina and dyspnoea. On examination you note a murmur at the right upper sternal border radiating to his neck. Which investigation is most likely to lead to a diagnosis?

   A. Chest X-ray
   B. Echocardiogram
   C. ECG
   D. Coronary angiography
   E. 24 hour ECG

17. A 42-year-old man presents with shortness of breath and haemoptysis. On examination you note a loud first heart sound and a rumbling mid-diastolic murmur at the apex. You request an echocardiogram and a chest X-ray. The following are all features of the chest X-ray in this condition EXCEPT?

   A. Large right atrium
   B. Large left atrium

   C. Kerley B lines
   D. Pulmonary venous hypertension
   E. Narrowed carina

18. A 55-year-old man presents to accident and emergency with shortness of breath and fatigue. On examination you note pitting oedema in both his lower limbs. You suspect heart failure. Which investigation is most likely to demonstrate the aetiology?

   A. Chest X-ray
   B. Echocardiogram
   C. ECG
   D. Coronary angiography
   E. 24-hour ECG

19. A 46-year-old woman presents with shortness of breath. She comments she feels particularly breathless when lying down and uses 5 pillows to sleep at night. On examination her pulse rate is regular at 122 beats/min and her blood pressure is stable at 122/65 mmHg. You note bi basal crackles when listening to her chest. You suspect heart failure and order a chest X-ray and echocardiogram. The following may all be features on her chest X-ray EXCEPT?

   A. Kerley B lines
   B. Hilar haziness
   C. Fluid in the left horizontal interlobar fissure
   D. Upper lobe venous engorgement
   E. Cardiomegaly

20. A 55-year-old banker is admitted to accident and emergency complaining of sudden onset shortness of breath. Following an echocardiogram he is diagnosed with heart failure. What is the most likely aetiological cause for cardiac failure in the western world?

   A. Ischaemic heart disease
   B. Hypertension
   C. Valvular dysfunction
   D. Cardiomyopathy
   E. Arrhythmia

36. A 31-year-old man presents with several months of shortness of breath and chest discomfort. An ECG shows evidence of T wave flattening. You request an echocardiogram which demonstrates dilated ventricles with global hypokinesis. What is the most likely diagnosis?

A. Dilated cardiomyopathy
B. Hypertrophic cardiomyopathy
C. Restrictive cardiomyopathy
D. Arrhythmogenic right ventricular cardiomyopathy
E. Myocarditis

37. A 27-year-old footballer presents with laboured breathing and chest pain. An ECG shows evidence of left ventricular hypertrophy. What is the most likely diagnosis?

A. Dilated cardiomyopathy
B. Hypertrophic cardiomyopathy
C. Restrictive cardiomyopathy
D. Arrhythmogenic right ventricular cardiomyopathy
E. Myocarditis

38. A 42-year-old woman presents with chest pain. She comments the pain is worse on inspiration but is relieved by leaning forward. Her past medical history includes breast carcinoma. What is the most likely diagnosis?

A. Acute pericarditis
B. Pericardial effusion
C. Pericardial tamponade
D. Constrictive pericarditis
E. Myocarditis

39. A 43-year-old obese woman with known breast cancer complains of shortness of breath. On examination you note soft heart sounds and obscuration of the apex beat. Which investigation is most likely to lead to a diagnosis?

A. Chest X-ray
B. Echocardiogram
C. ECG
D. Arterial blood gas
E. Coronary angiography

40. A 63-year-old retired doctor presents with nausea and headaches. His past medical history includes Type II diabetes mellitus. On examination you note his blood pressure is 165/76 mmHg. What is the next most appropriate step in management?

A. Beta Blockers
B. Calcium channel antagonists
C. ACE inhibitors
D. Diuretics
E. Alpha Blockers

41. A 65-year-old hypertensive patient is reviewed in the outpatient clinic complaining of visual disturbances. On examination you note flame shaped haemorrhages. What is the most likely diagnosis?

A. Grade 1 retinal disease
B. Grade 2 retinal disease
C. Grade 3 retinal disease
D. Grade 4 retinal disease
E. Grade 5 retinal disease

Extended matching questions

Theme: Chest pain

A. Angina pectoris
B. Pericarditis
C. Myocardial infarction
D. Aortic dissection
E. Reflux oesophagitis
F. Pulmonary infarct
G. Pneumonia
H. Costochondritis
I. Pneumothorax
J. Pulmonary embolus

For each scenario described below, choose the single most appropriate answer from the above list of options. Each option may be used once, more than once or not at all.

1. A middle aged man presenting with a central crushing chest pain on exercise but relieved by rest. ☐

2. Associated with central crushing chest pain which occurs at rest and may radiate to the jaw or arms. ☐

3. Severe tearing chest pain which may radiate to the back. ☐

4. Central chest discomfort which is sharp in nature with a tender area on palpation. ☐

5. Sharp chest pain aggravated by movement, respiration and changes in posture. ☐

Theme: **Drugs**

A. Propranolol
B. Nicorandil
C. Aspirin
D. Nifedipine
E. Captopril
F. Digoxin
G. Bisoprolol
H. Bendrofluazide
I. Clopidogrel
J. Simvastatin

For each scenario described below, choose the single most appropriate answer from the above list of options. Each option may be used once, more than once or not at all.

1. Used in the treatment of cardiac failure. Know to cause a persistent cough. ☐

2. Contraindicated in renal artery stenosis. ☐

3. Associated with bradycardia, headaches and fluid retention. ☐

4. First line management in acute coronary syndrome. ☐

5. Specifically contraindicated in asthmatics and individuals with peripheral vascular disease. ☐

Theme: **Clinical features of cardiac disease**

A. Aortic stenosis
B. Aortic regurgitation
C. Mitral stenosis
D. Mitral regurgitation
E. Infective endocarditis
F. Rheumatic fever
G. Tricuspid stenosis
H. Tricuspid regurgitation
I. Pulmonary hypertension
J. Pulmonary embolism

For each scenario described below, choose the single most appropriate answer from the above list of options. Each option may be used once, more than once or not at all.

1. A pansystolic murmur ausculated at the apex and radiating into the axilla. ☐

2. Associated with erythematous macules on the palms and haemorrhages under the nails. ☐

3. Associated with pink coloured rings on the trunk and subcutaneous nodules over the joints. ☐

4. Associated with a slow rising carotid pulse and ejection systolic murmur at the right upper sternal border. ☐

5. Known to cause a right parasternal heave and a loud pulmonary second sound. ☐

Gastroenterology and hepatobiliary medicine

Single best answer

1. A 32-year-old woman presents with epigastric pain. She comments that it is particularly worse at night. You refer her for a urea breath test which confirms the presence of *Helicobacter pylori*. The following are all proposed mechanisms of *Helicobacter pylori* pathogenesis EXCEPT?

   A. Increased parietal cell mass
   B. Increased somatostatin production
   C. Increased pepsinogen production
   D. Increased gastrin production
   E. Increased vacuolating toxin production

2. A 42-year-old alcoholic presents with heartburn. He comments it is aggravated by bending and lying down but relieved by drinking milk. What is the next most appropriate initial investigation?

   A. 24-hour oesophageal pH monitoring
   B. Barium swallow
   C. Upper gastrointestinal endoscopy
   D. Chest X-ray
   E. Abdominal X-ray

3. A 40-year-old obese city worker presents with heartburn. He comments that he tried 'Gaviscon' which barely relieved the pain. You suspect the diagnosis of gastro-oesophageal reflux disease. Which management plan would you instigate first?

   A. H$_2$ receptor antagonists
   B. Domperidone
   C. Nissen fundoplication
   D. Proton pump inhibitors
   E. Metoclopramide

4. A 35-year-old woman complains of difficulty in swallowing and weight loss. She comments she is unable to swallow both liquid and solid food. A barium swallow is performed which demonstrates a tapered lower end of her oesophagus. What is the most likely diagnosis?

   A. Achalasia
   B. Systemic sclerosis
   C. Diffuse oesophageal spasm
   D. Hiatus hernia
   E. Oesophageal carcinoma

5. A middle aged man presents complaining of swallowing difficulties and chest pain. A barium swallow is arranged which demonstrates a 'corkscrew' like appearance. What is the most likely diagnosis?

   A. Achalasia
   B. Systemic sclerosis
   C. Diffuse oesophageal spasm
   D. Hiatus hernia
   E. Oesophageal carcinoma

6. A 65-year-old Chinese man presents complaining of swallowing difficulties and weight loss of approximately 2 stones over a 1 month period. An upper gastrointestinal endoscopy is arranged which demonstrates evidence of a tumour mass. The following are all risk factors for squamous cell oesophageal carcinoma EXCEPT?

   A. Pickled vegetables
   B. Salted fish
   C. Smoking
   D. Alcohol
   E. Gastro-oesophageal reflux disease

7. A 42-year-old man presents with pain in his stomach after meals. An endoscopy is performed which shows evidence of gastritis and infection with *Helicobacter pylori*. What is the next most appropriate step in management?

   A. Metoclopramide, omeprazole and amoxicillin
   B. Omeprazole, metronidazole and cimetidine
   C. Omeprazole, metronidazole and clarithromycin
   D. Omeprazole, ranitidine and amoxicillin
   E. Domperidone, omeprazole and amoxicillin

8. A 56-year-old man presents with epigastric pain, vomiting and weight loss. He is a heavy drinker and admits to consuming half a bottle of vodka each day over a 10-year period. On examination you note a purple coloured peri orbital skin rash. What is the next most appropriate initial investigation?

   A. Abdominal CT scan
   B. Abdominal MRI scan
   C. Abdominal X-ray
   D. Upper gastrointestinal endoscopy
   E. Endoscopic ultrasound scan

9. A 42-year-old man presents with a 1 day history of haematemesis. On closer questioning he commented when he opens his bowels his motion looks like tar. What is the most likely aetiological cause for his symptoms?

   A. Mallory Weiss tear
   B. Reflux oesophagitis
   C. Gastric varices
   D. Oesophageal varices
   E. Peptic ulcer

10. A 21-year-old rugby player presents to accident and emergency with a 1 day history of haematemesis. He had recently been on a drinking binge following his team winning the local final. He comments the bleeding began after an episode of severe vomiting. An endoscopy is performed. What is the most likely diagnosis?

    A. Mallory Weiss tear
    B. Reflux oesophagitis

C. Gastric varices
D. Oesophageal varices
E. Peptic ulcer

11. A 75-year-old woman presents with a 1 day history of haematemesis. She comments she has been suffering from back pain for the past month for which she has been taking diclofenac as prescribed by her GP. What is the most likely aetiological cause for her symptoms?

    A. Mallory Weiss tear
    B. Reflux oesophagitis
    C. Peptic ulcer
    D. Gastric varices
    E. Oesophageal varices

12. While on call you are asked to see a patient who has just passed melaena. On examination you note he is drowsy with a pulse of 124 beats/min and blood pressure of 75/44 mmHg. Which management plan would you instigate first?

    A. Upper gastrointestinal endoscopy
    B. Colonoscopy
    C. Bloods for group and save and cross match
    D. Intravenous access and fluid resuscitation
    E. Laparotomy

13. You are a house officer in colorectal surgery when you are asked to see a patient who has had a fresh PR bleed. On examination the patient is haemodynamically stable. What is the next most appropriate step in management?

    A. Rectal examination
    B. Colonoscopy
    C. Sigmoidoscopy
    D. Proctoscopy
    E. Barium enema

14. A 45-year-old man presents with shortness of breath and fatigue. Routine blood investigations reveal a haemoglobin of 10.2 g/dl, a mean corpuscular volume (MCV) of 75 fl and a serum ferritin of 10 µg/l. What is the next most appropriate initial investigation?

A. Upper gastrointestinal endoscopy
B. Colonoscopy
C. Upper gastrointestinal endoscopy and colonoscopy
D. Barium meal and follow through
E. Mesenteric angiography

15. A 14-year-old girl presents with abdominal pain and diarrhoea. She is found to be iron and folate deficient on initial investigation. What is the most likely diagnosis?

A. Crohn's disease
B. Ulcerative colitis
C. Whipple's disease
D. Irritable bowel syndrome
E. Coeliac disease

16. A 15-year-old Irish boy is recently diagnosed with coeliac disease. The following are all features of the condition EXCEPT?

A. Sensitivity to alpha gliadin
B. Increased incidence in type I diabetes mellitus
C. Involvement of the jejunum
D. Elongation of small intestinal villi
E. Association with the haplotype DQ 2

17. A 19-year-old woman presents with abdominal pain and diarrhoea. She comments that there is a strong family history of coeliac disease. Which investigation is most likely to lead to a diagnosis?

A. Upper gastrointestinal endoscopy and distal duodenal biopsy
B. Full blood count
C. Small-bowel barium follow-through
D. Bone densitometry scan
E. Anti-reticulin antibodies

18. A 55-year-old man has recently undergone complicated small bowel surgery. He complains of producing loose stools which he describes as being offensive and difficult to flush. Which investigation is most likely to lead to a diagnosis?

A. Upper gastrointestinal endoscopy
B. Rectal examination
C. Hydrogen breath test
D. Barium meal
E. Abdominal CT scan

19. A 32-year-old woman is diagnosed with Crohn's disease. The following are all true statements with regards to Crohn's disease EXCEPT?

A. Smoking reduces the risk of developing the condition
B. Intestinal bacteria play a role in disease pathogenesis
C. The most common site affected is ileocaecal
D. Mutations within the NOD 2 gene are linked to the condition
E. Crohn's disease affects males and females equally

20. A 25-year-old woman is diagnosed with ulcerative colitis. The following are all features of ulcerative colitis EXCEPT?

A. Involvement of Th2 cells
B. Goblet cell depletion
C. Pseudo polyp formation
D. Skip lesions
E. Crypt abscess formation

21. A 21-year-old woman with ulcerative colitis presents with bloody diarrhoea opening her bowels up to 7 times per day. The following are all features of an acute attack of ulcerative colitis EXCEPT?

A. Bloody diarrhoea
B. Fever
C. Tachycardia
D. Raised erythrocyte sedimentation rate (ESR)
E. Tachypnoea

22. A 45-year-old smoker is recently diagnosed with inflammatory bowel disease. The following are all related to disease activity EXCEPT?

    A. Gall bladder calculi
    B. Venous thrombosis
    C. Uveitis
    D. Erythema nodosum
    E. Vasculitis

23. You are a house officer on call when you are asked to review a patient with Crohn's disease. The patient complains that his bowel frequency has increased from 2 times per day to 6 times per day. He also states he has severe lower abdominal pain. You bleep the on call gastroenterology registrar who tells you to take urgent bloods. The following are all markers of an acute exacerbation EXCEPT?

    A. Increased platelet count
    B. Increased C-reactive protein (CRP)
    C. Increased erythrocyte sedimentation rate (ESR)
    D. Low serum albumin
    E. Reduced plasma sodium

24. A middle aged man with ulcerative colitis is referred to accident and emergency by his GP with an acute flare opening his bowels 8 times per day. Routine blood investigations reveal a platelet count of $576 \times 10^9/l$ and C Reactive protein (CRP) of 156 mg/l. What is the next most appropriate step in management?

    A. Oral steroids
    B. Intravenous steroids
    C. Ciclosporin
    D. Mesalazine
    E. Azathioprine

25. A patient with Crohn's disease comes to see his GP. He is currently on mesalazine but has been experiencing an increase in bowel frequency and gradual onset of abdominal pain. What is the next most appropriate step in management?

    A. Steroids
    B. Ciclosporin
    C. Azathioprine

    D. Metronidazole
    E. Methotrexate

26. A middle aged woman with known Crohn's disease is worried about the complications of her condition. The following are all more common complications of Crohn's disease as opposed to ulcerative colitis EXCEPT?

    A. Colon cancer
    B. Erythema nodosum
    C. Stricture formation
    D. Abscess formation
    E. Fistulae formation

27. A 65-year-old woman presents with sudden onset left iliac fossa pain, fever and vomiting. Which investigation is most likely to lead to a diagnosis?

    A. Colonoscopy
    B. Abdominal ultrasound
    C. Abdominal and pelvic CT scan
    D. Abdominal X-ray
    E. White cell count and C-reactive protein (CRP)

28. A 72-year-old man presents to his GP complaining of not opening his bowels for the past 2 days. On examination you note slight abdominal distension but no evidence of abdominal tenderness. Rectal examination reveals hard impacted faeces. The following are all causes of constipation EXCEPT?

    A. Hypercalcaemia
    B. Hyperkalaemia
    C. Opiates
    D. Depression
    E. Low-fibre diet

29. A 65-year-old man presents with rectal bleeding and weight loss of approximately 2 stones over a 1 month period. A colonoscopy is performed which demonstrates a tumour mass in the sigmoid colon. Biopsies confirm

the presence of an adenocarcinoma. At subsequent resection the tumour had invaded the bowel wall with no involvement of adjacent lymph nodes. What is the Dukes' staging?

A. Duke's A colon cancer
B. Duke's B colon cancer
C. Duke's C1 colon cancer
D. Duke's C2 colon cancer
E. Duke's D colon cancer

30. A 55-year-old man presents with rectal bleeding and abdominal discomfort. A colonoscopy is performed which reveals the presence of a tumour in the sigmoid colon. Further assessment and staging confirms a colonic adenocarcinoma with probable local lymph node involvement. What is the next most appropriate step in management?

A. Surgery
B. Chemotherapy
C. Surgery and adjuvant chemotherapy
D. Radiotherapy
E. Palliative treatment

31. A 55-year-old woman presents with abdominal pain and diarrhoea. She notices fresh red blood in the toilet pan when she opens her bowels. She smokes 25 cigarettes a day since the age of 30 and drinks 8 units of alcohol a week. Her mother was diagnosed with bowel cancer at 40 years of age. She enjoys eating steak but admits she does not have a taste for fruit or vegetables. You arrange a barium study which confirms the presence of a colonic tumour. What is the most likely aetiological cause for her tumour?

A. Poor diet
B. Smoking
C. Alcohol
D. Family history
E. Age

32. A 32-year-old woman with severe Crohn's disease underwent a subtotal colectomy with ileostomy formation. She comes to the GP complaining of increased stoma output. She comments she is emptying her bag up to 6 times per day and that the contents are loose and watery. What is the next most appropriate initial investigation?

A. Ileoscopy
B. Barium meal and follow through
C. Hydrogen breath test
D. Abdominal CT scan
E. Stool culture

33. A 65-year-old woman is on long term total parenteral nutrition (TPN) via a Hickman line following a small bowel resection. While on call you are asked to review the patient as she has a temperature of 38.5°C. What is the next most appropriate step in management?

A. Peripheral blood cultures and continue TPN
B. Hickman line blood cultures and continue TPN
C. Peripheral and Hickman line blood cultures and continue TPN
D. Peripheral and Hickman line blood cultures and stop TPN
E. Paracetamol as required and recheck temperature in 30 minutes.

34. A 65-year-old man presents with right-sided abdominal pain. On examination you note a moderately enlarged liver and a yellow discoloration of his skin and eyes. What is the next most appropriate initial investigation?

A. Abdominal ultrasound scan
B. Endoscopic retrograde cholangiopancreatography (ERCP)
C. Viral markers
D. Liver biopsy
E. Magnetic resonance cholangiopancreatography (MRCP)

35. A 23-year-old South American man presents with abdominal pain and diarrhoea over a 3 day period followed by jaundice. He comments that his urine appears darker than usual but says he is drinking plenty of water. He has recently travelled to Lima to see his family. What is the most likely diagnosis?

    A. Hepatitis D
    B. Hepatitis A
    C. Hepatitis E
    D. Hepatitis B
    E. Hepatitis C

36. A 35-year-old intravenous drug abuser presents with abdominal pain and nausea. He also comments his joints feel stiff. Routine blood investigations reveal an alanine aminotransferase (ALT) of 1278 U/l, an aspartate aminotransferase (AST) of 990 U/l and a bilirubin of 65 micromol/l. What is the most likely diagnosis?

    A. Hepatitis D
    B. Hepatitis A
    C. Hepatitis B
    D. Hepatitis E
    E. Hepatitis C

37. A 56-year-old Egyptian woman presents with fatigue and nausea. She complains that her skin feels itchy and that she has noticed blood when she passes urine. On examination you note a yellow tinge to her skin and sclera. What is the most likely diagnosis?

    A. Hepatitis A
    B. Hepatitis D
    C. Hepatitis B
    D. Hepatitis E
    E. Hepatitis C

38. A 32-year-old man presents with abdominal pain, diarrhoea and jaundice. He has recently been to Dubai with his wife. He comments the best thing about Dubai is the seafood. What is the next most appropriate step in management?

    A. Alpha interferon
    B. Lamivudine
    C. Ribavirin
    D. Watchful waiting
    E. Pegylated alpha-interferon

39. A 32-year-old man presents to accident and emergency following a paracetamol overdose. Routine blood investigations reveal an alanine aminotransferase (ALT) of 1800 U/l and a prothrombin time of 42 seconds. On examination he appears drowsy and is not communicative. What is his grade of encephalopathy?

    A. Grade 1 encephalopathy
    B. Grade 2 encephalopathy
    C. Grade 3 encephalopathy
    D. Grade 4 encephalopathy
    E. Grade 5 encephalopathy

40. A middle aged woman with autoimmune thyroiditis presents with nausea and fatigue. On examination you note jaundice and spider naevi. Which investigation is most likely to lead to a diagnosis?

    A. Abdominal ultrasound
    B. High titres of antinuclear antibodies
    C. High serum ferritin levels
    D. Hepatitis B testing
    E. IgM levels

41. A 43-year-old man with a long-standing history of alcohol abuse presents to accident and emergency with haematemesis. On examination you note a liver flap and evidence of moderate hepatomegaly. You suspect a diagnosis of cirrhosis. Which investigation is most likely to assess the patient's liver function?

    A. Liver biochemistry
    B. Serum electrolytes
    C. Serum alpha fetoprotein
    D. Prothrombin time
    E. Hepatitis serology

42. A middle aged man with alcoholic cirrhosis comes to see his GP. He is worried about his overall survival rate. You explain to him his prognosis is dependent on a variety of factors. The following are all variables important in assessing the prognosis of liver disease EXCEPT?

  A. Encephalopathy
  B. Serum albumin
  C. Serum bilirubin
  D. Prothrombin time
  E. Serum transaminases

43. A 25-year-old city worker presents with a 2-day history of haematemesis following a weekend of binge drinking. Which management plan would you instigate first?

  A. Upper gastrointestinal endoscopy
  B. Intravenous terlipressin
  C. Laparotomy
  D. Transjugular intrahepatic portosystemic shunting (TIPS)
  E. Sucralfate

44. A 65-year-old man presents with loss of appetite and weight loss. On examination you note obvious ascites. You perform an ascitic tap which demonstrates the presence of an exudate. The following are all examples of an exudate EXCEPT?

  A. Infection
  B. Meig's syndrome
  C. Pancreatitis
  D. Budd Chiari syndrome
  E. Myxoedema

45. A middle aged man is diagnosed with liver cirrhosis secondary to chronic alcohol abuse. On examination you note dullness in his flanks. Which management plan would you instigate first?

  A. Paracentesis
  B. Sodium restriction alone
  C. Sodium restriction and diuretics

  D. Transjugular intrahepatic portosystemic shunting (TIPS)
  E. Albumin infusion

46. A 35-year-old man with alcoholic cirrhosis complains of abdominal discomfort. On examination you note the presence of ascites and notable peritonism. Routine blood investigations reveal a white cell count of $23 \times 10^9/l$ and C Reactive protein (CRP) of 107 mg/l. What is the most likely aetiological cause for his symptoms?

  A. *Staphylococcus aureus*
  B. *Escherichia coli*
  C. *Enterococcus faecalis*
  D. *Proteus mirabilis*
  E. *Staphylococcus epidermidis*

47. A middle aged man presents to accident and emergency with confusion. His wife comments he doesn't appear to be his usual self and that he has been drinking excessively for many years. On examination you note a liver flap and a sweet smell on his breath. How would you usually make the diagnosis leading to his confusion?

  A. Electroencephalography (EEG)
  B. Head CT scan
  C. Abdominal CT scan
  D. Abdominal ultrasound
  E. Clinical assessment

48. A 47-year-old woman complains that her skin is feeling itchy and her stools are difficult to flush. On examination she has moderate hepatomegaly and investigations demonstrate a raised serum alkaline phosphatase. Which investigation is most likely to lead to a diagnosis?

  A. Serum IgM
  B. Serum aspartate aminotransferase (AST)
  C. Serum bilirubin
  D. Serum antimitochondrial antibodies (AMAs)
  E. Antinuclear factor

49. A middle aged man complains of malaise and arthropathy. He is a newly diagnosed diabetic and on examination has evidence of hepatomegaly. Which investigation is most likely to lead to a diagnosis?
    A. Serum aspartate aminotransferase (AST)
    B. Serum bilirubin
    C. Serum albumin
    D. International normalised ratio (INR)
    E. Serum ferritin

50. A middle aged woman with suspected alcoholic liver disease is referred for a liver biopsy. The histology report states that there is necrosis of the liver cells and infiltration of leucocytes with the presence of mallory bodies within the hepatocytes. What is the next most appropriate step in management?
    A. Liver transplant
    B. Steroids
    C. Stop alcohol completely
    D. Continue alcohol in moderation
    E. Multivitamins and nutritional support

51. A 65-year-old man presents with weight loss and abdominal pain. On examination you note evidence of ascites. Routine blood investigations reveal a markedly raised alpha fetoprotein level and deranged liver function tests. What is the next most appropriate initial investigation?
    A. Abdominal X-ray
    B. Abdominal MRI scan
    C. Liver biopsy
    D. Ultrasound
    E. Hepatic angiogram

52. A 24-year-old obese woman presents to accident and emergency with sudden onset severe right upper quadrant pain. On examination you note notable tenderness in the right upper quadrant with guarding. Which investigation is most likely to lead to a diagnosis?
    A. White cell count
    B. C-reactive protein (CRP)
    C. Liver function tests
    D. Abdominal X-ray
    E. Abdominal ultrasound

53. A 42-year-old chronic alcohol abuser presents with epigastric pain radiating to his back. Blood investigations reveal an amylase of 1000 U/l. The following are all common complications of the above condition EXCEPT?
    A. Hypoglycaemia
    B. Hypocalcaemia
    C. Renal failure
    D. Shock
    E. Respiratory failure

54. A middle aged woman with chronic alcohol dependency presents with abdominal pain and weight loss. She comments her stools are difficult to flush. What is the next most appropriate initial investigation?
    A. Erect chest X-ray
    B. Abdominal X-ray
    C. Endoscopic retrograde cholangiopancreatography (ERCP)
    D. Abdominal CT scan
    E. Magnetic resonance cholangiopancreatography (MRCP)

55. An 85-year-old frail woman presents with abdominal pain and weight loss of over 2 stone in a 1 month period. An abdominal ultrasound scan is performed which confirms the diagnosis as pancreatic cancer with liver metastases. What is the next most appropriate step in management?
    A. Surgery
    B. Palliative therapy
    C. Radiotherapy
    D. Chemotherapy
    E. Surgery and chemotherapy

Extended matching questions

Theme: **Hepatobiliary disorders**

A. Wilson's disease
B. Alpha 1 antitrypsin deficiency
C. Hepatitis A
D. Cirrhosis
E. Hepatitis E
F. Primary sclerosing cholangitis
G. Haemochromatosis
H. Hepatocellular carcinoma
I. Hepatitis C
J. Primary biliary cirrhosis

For each scenario described below, choose the single most appropriate answer from the above list of options. Each option may be used once, more than once or not at all.

1. An autosomal recessive disorder associated with the C282Y mutation on chromosome 6. ☐

2. An autosomal recessive disorder associated with cirrhotic changes and the presence of periodic-acid-Schiff-positive staining globules within hepatocytes. ☐

3. A condition known to primarily affect middle aged women resulting in pruritus, jaundice, xanthomas and bone disease. ☐

4. An autosomal recessive disorder known to cause basal ganglia damage and renal failure best managed by trientene. ☐

5. A condition associated with abdominal pain, jaundice and cirrhosis seen in individuals with inflammatory bowel disease. ☐

Theme: **Gastrointestinal bleeding**

A. Mallory Weiss tear
B. Angiodysplasia
C. Haemorrhoids
D. Colon cancer
E. Duodenal ulcer
F. Oesophageal varices
G. Reflux oesophagitis
H. Gastritis
I. Gastric erosions
J. Anal fissure

For each scenario described below, choose the single most appropriate answer from the above list of options. Each option may be used once, more than once or not at all.

1. A middle aged woman presenting with spots of bright red blood on the toilet paper after passing stool. ☐

2. A university student presenting with haematemesis following a period of vigorous vomiting. ☐

3. A cause of iron deficiency anaemia affecting the colon, caecum or terminal ileum in individuals with aortic stenosis. ☐

4. Associated with heartburn and odynophagia. ☐

5. Associated with epigastric discomfort which is typically relieved by food and caused by infection with a gram negative bacterium. ☐

Theme: **Drugs**

A. Omeprazole
B. Aspirin
C. Penicillamine
D. Acamprosate
E. Mesalazine
F. Steroids
G. Nifedipine
H. Cisapride
I. Chlordiazepoxide
J. Alpha interferon

For each scenario described below, choose the single most appropriate answer from the above list of options. Each option may be used once, more than once or not at all.

1. A chronic alcohol user who has had three recent admissions to hospital following an alcoholic 'binge'. He is demanding medication to help prevent him drink again. ☐

2. A patient with known ulcerative colitis admitted to accident and emergency following an acute flare. ☐

3. A 65-year-old man with a history of stroke presenting with an episode of haematemesis. ☐

4. A middle aged obese man presenting with indigestion following consumption of spicy foods. ☐

5. A 23-year-old female presenting with abdominal discomfort and diarrhoea. A colonoscopy and subsequent biopsies demonstrates evidence of transmural inflammation with non-caseating granulomas. ☐

Theme: **Dysphagia**

A. Achalasia
B. Oesophageal carcinoma
C. Benign oesophageal stricture
D. Oesophagitis
E. Pharyngeal pouch
F. Oesophageal pouch
G. Oesophageal web
H. Foreign body
I. Candida
J. Cytomegalovirus

For each scenario described below, choose the single most appropriate answer from the above list of options. Each option may be used once, more than once or not at all.

1. A patient presenting with swallowing difficulties and oral discomfort following a recent renal transplant. ☐

2. Associated with swallowing difficulties, persistent coughing and iron-deficiency anaemia. ☐

3. Associated with regurgitation of food as a result of abnormal motility of the cricopharyngeus muscle and inferior constrictor. ☐

4. A middle aged man presenting with swallowing difficulties of both liquid and solid food following recent sclerotherapy of oesophageal varices. ☐

5. Associated with intermittent dysphagia of both liquid and solid food. A chest radiograph demonstrates evidence of a fluid level behind the heart. ☐

Theme: **Gastroenteritis**

A. Clostridium perfringens
B. Campylobacter
C. Bacillus cereus
D. Vibrio cholerae
E. Escherichia coli
F. Yersinia enterocolitica
G. Salmonella
H. Staphylococcus aureus
I. Vibrio parahaemolyticus
J. Norwalk virus

For each scenario described below, choose the single most appropriate answer from the above list of options. Each option may be used once, more than once or not at all.

1. Known to cause nausea, vomiting and diarrhoea approximately 1 to 6 hours following ingestion of contaminated dairy products or cold meat. ☐

2. Associated with vomiting and later diarrhoea following consumption of reheated rice. ☐

3. Associated with abdominal pain, diarrhoea and rectal bleeding following consumption of contaminated poultry. ☐

4. Known to cause bloody diarrhoea within 1 to 2 days of consuming contaminated meat. The use of antibiotics is specifically contraindicated. ☐

5. Associated with diarrhoea, abdominal pain and bloody stools following contact with infected animals or ice cream. ☐

SURGERY – QUESTIONS

9. Surgical emergencies   73

10. Hernia   77

11. Vascular surgery   79

12. Breast disease   83

13. Orthopaedics   87

14. Ear, nose and throat   91

15. Trauma   95

16. Urology   99

17. Perioperative care   103

18. Gastrointestinal surgery   105

Single best answer

1. A 32-year-old man presents with a 2-day history of sudden onset pain in the right iliac fossa. On examination you note guarding and rebound tenderness localised to an area approximately one third of the distance from the anterior superior iliac spine and umbilicus on the right side of his abdomen. What is being described here?

    A. Grey Turner's sign
    B. Cullen's sign
    C. McBurney's point
    D. Rovsing's sign
    E. Murphy's sign

2. A 26-year-old woman presents with sudden onset right iliac fossa pain. On examination you note that when pressure is applied to her left iliac fossa the patient complains of increased pain in her lower right side. What is being described here?

    A. Grey Turner's sign
    B. Cullen's sign
    C. McBurney's point
    D. Rovsing's sign
    E. Murphy's sign

3. A 32-year-old woman presents with lower right sided abdominal pain. She describes the pain as initially being centralised and associated with nausea. Routine blood investigations reveal a white cell count of $23 \times 10^9/l$. A urine dipstick reveals 3+ leucocytes. Which investigation is least useful in establishing the diagnosis?

    A. Abdominal X-ray
    B. Abdominal ultrasound
    C. Pregnancy test
    D. Abdominal CT scan
    E. Pelvic ultrasound

4. A 42-year-old man presents with generalised abdominal pain and vomiting. He comments he has not opened his bowels for the past 2 days. On examination you note severe abdominal distension and tinkling bowel sounds. An abdominal X-ray is ordered which reveals distended loops of small bowel. What is the next most appropriate step in management?

    A. Nasogastric decompression and normal saline IV
    B. Surgery
    C. Nasogastric decompression
    D. Nasogastric decompression and dextrose IV
    E. Normal saline IV

5. A 35-year-old chronic alcohol abuser complains of upper abdominal pain radiating to his back. On examination you note tenderness and guarding in the epigastrium. Which investigation is most likely to lead to a definitive diagnosis?

    A. Abdominal CT scan
    B. Abdominal X-ray
    C. Chest X-ray
    D. Abdominal ultrasound
    E. Liver function tests

6. A 42-year-old man presents with upper abdominal pain. Routine blood investigations reveal an amylase of 1050 IU/l. A diagnosis of acute pancreatitis is made. The following are all indicators of severity of pancreatitis EXCEPT?

    A. Age greater than 55 years
    B. Leucocyte count greater than $15 \times 10^9/l$
    C. Blood urea greater than 16 mmol/l
    D. Serum calcium less than 2 mmol/l
    E. Arterial PO_2 less than 9 kPa

7. A 32-year-old man presents with severe abdominal pain radiating to his back. On examination you note notable tenderness and guarding in the epigastric region. In addition you note evidence of bruising around the umbilicus. What is the term most likely used to describe this finding?

   A. Grey Turner's sign
   B. Cullen's sign
   C. McBurney's point
   D. Rovsing's sign
   E. Murphy's sign

8. A 42-year-old man is diagnosed with acute pancreatitis. The following are all complications of acute pancreatitis EXCEPT?

   A. Ascites
   B. Fat necrosis
   C. Muscle wasting
   D. Portal vein thrombosis
   E. Paralytic ileus

9. A 42-year-old man presents with severe colicky pain in his right loin radiating to his groin. On examination you note tenderness in the right loin. A urine dipstick is performed which is positive for blood. What is the next most appropriate initial investigation?

   A. Abdominal ultrasound
   B. Abdominal X-ray
   C. Abdominal CT scan
   D. 24-hour urine collection
   E. Intravenous urogram

10. A middle aged obese gentleman presents with severe right upper quadrant abdominal pain after a Chinese take away. On examination you note tenderness in his epigastrium and right upper quadrant. Which investigation is most likely to establish the actual diagnosis?

    A. White cell count
    B. Abdominal ultrasound
    C. Liver function tests
    D. Abdominal X-ray
    E. Serum amylase

11. A 65-year-old hypertensive patient presents to accident and emergency with sudden onset central abdominal pain radiating to his back. On examination you note evidence of generalised severe abdominal tenderness and a pulsatile mass. Routine observations reveal a pulse rate of 129 beats/min and blood pressure of 75/40 mmHg. What is the next most appropriate step in management?

    A. IV access and fluid resuscitation with Gelofusine
    B. IV access and blood resuscitation
    C. Abdominal CT scan
    D. Abdominal ultrasound
    E. Immediate transfer for surgery while simultaneously performing resuscitation

12. A 55-year-old woman presents with pain and numbness in her right leg. Her past medical history includes atrial fibrillation. On examination of her right leg you note absent pulses, pallor and a reduction in temperature as compared to her left limb. Routine observations reveal an irregular pulse of 125 beats/min, blood pressure of 105/65 mmHg and oxygen saturation of 96% on room air. Following initial resuscitation what is the next most appropriate step in management?

    A. ECG
    B. Digoxin
    C. Embolectomy
    D. Intravenous fluids
    E. Oxygen

13. An elderly patient presents with left iliac fossa pain and vomiting. On examination you note evidence of tenderness in the left iliac fossa and peritonism. Routine blood investigations demonstrate a white cell count of $22 \times 10^9/l$. What is the most likely diagnosis?

    A. Diverticulitis
    B. Ulcerative colitis
    C. Sigmoid volvulus
    D. Small bowel obstruction
    E. Large bowel obstruction

14. A middle aged obese gentleman presents with right upper quadrant pain. Abdominal examination reveals evidence of severe tenderness in the right upper quadrant. Routine observations reveal a temperature of 38.5°C. Blood tests confirm a white cell count of 16×10^9/l and C-reactive protein (CRP) of 135 mg/l. What is the most likely diagnosis?

   A. Pancreatitis
   B. Large bowel obstruction
   C. Large bowel perforation
   D. Cholecystitis
   E. Hepatitis

15. A 35-year-old woman presents with lower left-sided abdominal discomfort that is severe in nature. She denies any gastrointestinal symptoms. Abdominal examination confirms evidence of lower abdominal tenderness. Routine blood investigations reveal a normal white cell count and C-reactive protein. Serum β HCG is negative. What is the most likely diagnosis?

   A. Diverticulitis
   B. Ovarian cyst
   C. Uterine cyst
   D. Sigmoid volvulus
   E. Ectopic pregnancy

16. A 15-year-old boy presents with sudden onset severe pain in his left scrotum and vomiting. On examination you note marked tenderness on palpation. A urine dipstick proves normal. What is the most likely diagnosis?

   A. Epididymitis
   B. Hydrocele
   C. Orchitis
   D. Appendicitis
   E. Testicular torsion

17. A 25-year-old sexually active male presents with scrotal swelling and pain. On examination you note evidence of scrotal erythema. A urine dipstick proves positive for leucocytes. What is the most likely diagnosis?

   A. Epididymitis
   B. Hydrocele
   C. Urinary tract infection
   D. Appendicitis
   E. Testicular torsion

Extended matching questions

Theme: Acute abdomen

   A. Appendicitis
   B. Pancreatitis
   C. Renal colic
   D. Abdominal aortic aneurysm
   E. Thoracic aortic aneurysm
   F. Dissecting aortic aneurysm
   G. Peptic ulcer disease
   H. Bowel obstruction
   I. Biliary colic
   J. Perforated viscus

For each scenario described below, choose the single most appropriate answer from the above list of options. Each option may be used once, more than once or not at all.

1. Associated with colicky abdominal pain, vomiting and absent bowel movement. ☐

2. A patient presenting with generalized abdominal tenderness with evidence of free gas on an erect chest X-ray. ☐

3. Associated with colicky abdominal pain in the left flank with radiation to the groin. Abdominal signs are usually minimal. The pain may be so severe as to interrupt one's breath. ☐

4. A medical student presents with severe upper abdominal tenderness and a serum amylase greater than 4 times the normal limit. ☐

5. Associated with sudden onset severe tearing chest pain radiating to the back. A chest X-ray demonstrates evidence of a widened mediastinum. ☐

Single best questions

1. A 25-year-old weight lifter presents with a lump near the right side of his groin. On examination you note that the lump reduces upwards and laterally and moves downwards and medially on release. In addition you note the lump is controlled by pressure over the deep ring. What is the most likely diagnosis?

   A. Indirect inguinal hernia
   B. Direct inguinal hernia
   C. Femoral hernia
   D. Richter's hernia
   E. Sliding hernia

2. A 53-year-old man presents with a lump near his groin. On examination you note it reduces immediately on lying down and reaches full size immediately on standing. You ask the patient to cough and notice it protrudes straight. It is not controlled by pressure over the deep ring. What is the most likely diagnosis?

   A. Indirect inguinal hernia
   B. Direct inguinal hernia
   C. Femoral hernia
   D. Richter's hernia
   E. Sliding hernia

3. A 26-year-old man is diagnosed with an indirect inguinal hernia. The following are all common features of an indirect inguinal hernia EXCEPT?

   A. Descent into the scrotum
   B. Strangulation
   C. At operation, it is seen to arise laterally to the inferior epigastric vessels
   D. At operation, it is seen to arise medially to the inferior epigastric vessels
   E. The sac typically has a narrow neck

4. A 35-year-old woman presents with a lump in her groin. On examination you note the lump is below and lateral to the pubic tubercle. What is the most likely diagnosis?

   A. Indirect inguinal hernia
   B. Direct inguinal hernia
   C. Femoral hernia
   D. Richter's hernia
   E. Sliding hernia

5. A 25-year-old woman complains of pain at the navel. On examination you note an obvious swelling at the site of the umbilicus, which she says has been present since birth. What is the most likely diagnosis?

   A. Umbilical hernia
   B. Femoral hernia
   C. Richter's hernia
   D. Sliding hernia
   E. Para-umbilical hernia

6. A 43-year-old man presents with epigastric pain and associated nausea. On examination you note a palpable swelling in the midline which is tender and irreducible. What is the most likely diagnosis?

   A. Epigastric hernia
   B. Umbilical hernia
   C. Para-umbilical hernia
   D. Richter's hernia
   E. Sliding hernia

7. A 25-year-old man is diagnosed with an incisional hernia following a laparotomy for large bowel obstruction. The following are all

preoperative risk factors for incisional hernia formation EXCEPT?

A. Age

B. Diabetes

C. Malnutrition

D. Gender

E. Jaundice

8. A 42-year-old woman presents with a lump at the lateral edge of the rectus sheath. What is the most likely diagnosis?

A. Epigastric hernia

B. Umbilical hernia

C. Spigelian hernia

D. Para-umbilical hernia

E. Richter's hernia

9. A 65-year-old woman presents with a 2-day history of abdominal discomfort and vomiting. In addition she complains of right-sided hip pain. An abdominal X-ray is ordered which confirms evidence of small bowel obstruction. She undergoes an emergency laparotomy. What is the most likely diagnosis?

A. Epigastric hernia

B. Obturator hernia

C. Umbilical hernia

D. Para-umbilical hernia

E. Richter's hernia

Extended matching questions

Theme: **Hernia**

A. Inguinal

B. Pantaloon

C. Para-umbilical

D. Sciatic

E. Cooper's

F. Incisional

G. Richter's

H. Littre's

I. Spigelian

J. Diaphragmatic

For each scenario described below, choose the single most appropriate answer from the above list of options. Each option may be used once, more than once or not at all.

1. Associated with abdominal pain, notable distension and vomiting. It may result in perforation of the bowel. ☐

2. Seen commonly in newborn babies where typically the left side of the chest is occupied by bowel. ☐

3. A hernia occurring through a part of the abdominal wall between the lateral border of the rectus abdominis and linea semilunaris typically diagnosed by ultrasound. ☐

4. A combined indirect and direct hernia whereby the hernial sac protrudes on either side of the inferior epigastric vessels. ☐

5. A lump located near the groin which protrudes straight on coughing and is not controlled by pressure over the deep ring. ☐

Single best answer

1. **A middle aged man presents with sudden onset back pain and difficulty in swallowing. On examination his blood pressure is stable at 126/76 mmHg and pulse rate regular at 82 beats/min. What is the most likely diagnosis?**

   A. Thoracic aortic aneurysm

   B. False aneurysm

   C. Abdominal aortic aneurysm

   D. Mycotic aneurysm

   E. Popliteal aneurysm

2. **A 42-year-old woman presents with sudden onset abdominal and back pain. An abdominal CT scan is arranged which confirms the presence of an abdominal aortic aneurysm. The patient is referred for surgery. Post-operatively the patient complains of weakness in her lower limbs. What is the most likely aetiological cause for this weakness?**

   A. Vertebral artery damage

   B. Cervical radicular artery damage

   C. Thoracic radicular artery damage

   D. Iliac artery damage

   E. Artery of Adamkiewicz damage

3. **A 35-year-old smoker comes to see his GP for a routine check up. On examination the GP notes a pulsatile mass in his abdomen. An abdominal CT scan is arranged which confirms the presence of an abdominal aortic aneurysm. The following are all true of abdominal aortic aneurysms EXCEPT?**

   A. Males are more likely to be affected than females

   B. Repair is advised for aneurysms over 5.5 cm in size

   C. The abdominal aorta is considered aneurysmal if its diameter exceeds 5 cm

   D. A positive family history is a risk factor for aneurysm formation

   E. Smoking is associated with aneurysm formation

4. **A 36-year-old man presents to his GP. On abdominal examination the GP notes a pulsatile mass. The GP suspects an abdominal aortic aneurysm. What is the next most appropriate initial investigation?**

   A. Abdominal X-ray

   B. Abdominal ultrasound

   C. Abdominal MRI scan

   D. Abdominal CT scan

   E. Echocardiography

5. **A 45-year-old man presents to accident and emergency complaining of severe centralised abdominal pain. He comments the pain came on suddenly and is radiating to his back. On examination you note severe tenderness in his epigastric region. Routine observations demonstrate a blood pressure of 75/45 mmHg and pulse rate of 147 beats/min. You suspect a diagnosis of a ruptured abdominal aortic aneurysm. The following are all true with regards to ruptured abdominal aortic aneurysms EXCEPT?**

   A. Abdominal CT scan with intravenous contrast should only be performed if the patient is stable

   B. Emergency surgery is needed

   C. Blood should be taken for cross match

   D. Urgent fluid resuscitation is needed to maintain a systolic blood pressure of at least 140 mmHg

   E. Acute pancreatitis is a possible differential diagnosis

Extended matching questions

Theme: Vascular disorders

A. Abdominal aortic aneurysm

B. Thoracic aortic aneurysm

C. Dissecting aortic aneurysm

D. Compartment syndrome

E. Thromboangiitis obliterans

F. Raynaud's disease

G. Raynaud's phenomenon

H. Varicose veins

I. Thrombophlebitis migrans

J. Deep venous thrombosis

For each scenario described below, choose the single most appropriate answer from the above list of options. Each option may be used once, more than once or not at all.

1. Typically affects young men who smoke. The condition is progressive unless one stops smoking. ☐

2. A disease of young women whereby arteries of the fingers and toes are reactive and enter spasm in response to the cold. There is often no underlying vascular disease. ☐

3. Inflammation of a vein associated with pain, tenderness and redness. There is often an association with connective tissue disease. ☐

4. Associated with a pulsatile mass on abdominal examination with possible evidence of calcification on abdominal X-ray. ☐

5. A condition associated with severe tearing central chest pain radiating to the back. Blood pressure is often unequal in both arms. ☐

Single best answer

1. A 35-year-old woman presents to her GP complaining of a lump in the upper outer quadrant of her right breast. She comments the lump becomes particularly tender before the start of her menstrual cycle. What is the most likely diagnosis?

   A. Localised fibroadenosis
   B. Fibroadenoma
   C. Cyst
   D. Fat necrosis
   E. Carcinoma

2. A 31-year-old woman presents complaining of a lump in her left breast. On examination you note the lump is non-tender, rubbery and fairly mobile. What is the most likely diagnosis?

   A. Localised fibroadenosis
   B. Cyst
   C. Fat necrosis
   D. Fibroadenoma
   E. Carcinoma

3. A 55-year-old woman presents with a lump on her right breast. On examination you note the lump is tense and mobile. On fine-needle aspiration you note the production of a straw-coloured fluid. What is the most likely diagnosis?

   A. Localised fibroadenosis
   B. Fibroadenoma
   C. Fat necrosis
   D. Carcinoma
   E. Cyst

4. A 34-year-old woman smoker presents with a green-coloured discharge from both her nipples. On examination you note evidence of nipple retraction and breast lumpiness. What is the most likely diagnosis?

   A. Mammary duct ectasia
   B. Duct papilloma
   C. Galactorrhoea
   D. Duct carcinoma
   E. Paget's disease

5. A middle aged woman presents with a serous discharge from her right nipple. On examination the breast appears normal but on deep palpation the discharge is produced. What is the most likely diagnosis?

   A. Mammary duct ectasia
   B. Duct papilloma
   C. Galactorrhoea
   D. Duct carcinoma
   E. Paget's disease

6. A 55-year-old woman presents with a painless lump in her right breast. On general examination you note enlargement of her right axillary lymph nodes. You suspect the diagnosis of breast cancer. The following are all high risk factors for breast cancer EXCEPT?

   A. Age greater than 50
   B. A north European origin
   C. Age less than 35 years
   D. Nulliparity
   E. Previous history of breast cancer

7. A 57-year-old woman is recently diagnosed with breast cancer. Her GP comments she was at high risk due to her strong family history of breast cancer. The GP explains that particular chromosomes are linked to the condition. Which chromosome is most likely to be associated with breast cancer?

   A. Chromosome 14
   B. Chromosome 15
   C. Chromosome 16
   D. Chromosome 17
   E. Chromosome 18

8. A 45-year-old woman is concerned about developing breast cancer. She comes to see you asking when she will be called for a 'screening mammogram'. At what ages do women in the UK undergo screening as part of a National Programme?

   A. 50–64
   B. 45–59
   C. 55–69
   D. 46–60
   E. 56–70

9. A 54-year-old woman presents with a 5 cm lump in her right breast. On examination you note the presence of fixed right-sided axillary nodes. There are no palpable supraclavicular or infraclavicular nodes. You refer her for tissue biopsies. The histology report confirms the presence of a moderately differentiated adenocarcinoma with no evidence of distant metastasis. According to the International Union against Cancer what is the most likely staging classification of this presentation?

   A. Stage 1
   B. Stage 2
   C. Stage 3
   D. Stage 4
   E. Stage 5

10. A 52-year-old woman presents with a lump approximately 4 cm in size in her right breast. On examination you note no palpable nodes in her axilla, supraclavicular or infraclavicular region. Wide local excision and axillary node clearance confirm the presence of a well differentiated cancer with no evidence of lymph node involvement. According to the International Union against Cancer what is the most likely 5-year survival rate for this presentation?

    A. 84%
    B. 71%
    C. 59%
    D. 48%
    E. 18%

11. A 64-year-old woman presents with a lump in her left breast. On examination the lump is non-tender and painless. In addition you note dimpling of the skin and retraction of her left nipple. You refer her for urgent tissue biopsies which confirm the presence of an adenocarcinoma with associated fibrosis. Having explained the diagnosis you explain that this tumour is the most common type of tumour to affect women. What is the most likely diagnosis?

    A. Ductal
    B. Lobular
    C. Medullary
    D. Colloid
    E. Sarcoma

12. A 28-year-old woman presents with a lump on her right breast. On examination you note the lump is tense, discrete and mobile. You suspect the possibility of a breast cyst. Which investigation is the most appropriate in this scenario?

    A. Mammography
    B. CT chest scan
    C. MRI chest scan
    D. Ultrasound
    E. Chest X-ray

13. A 39-year-old woman is diagnosed with left-sided breast cancer. The tumour is confirmed as an oestrogen-receptor-negative, well differentiated adenocarcinoma approximately

6.5 cm in size. There is involvement of ipsilateral axillary nodes but no evidence of distant metastasis. She is referred to a breast surgeon who explains possible treatment options. What is the next most appropriate step in management?

A. Neoadjuvant chemotherapy and surgical excision with axillary clearance
B. Primary surgical excision of tumour without axillary dissection
C. Radiotherapy
D. Tamoxifen
E. Herceptin

14. A middle aged woman presents with a scaly red coloured rash affecting her right nipple and areola. She comments it is sore and has a tendency to bleed. What is the most likely diagnosis?

A. Mammary duct ectasia
B. Duct papilloma
C. Galactorrhoea
D. Duct carcinoma
E. Paget's disease

15. A 52-year-old woman presents with a fairly large painless lump in her left breast. On examination you note it appears fleshy and has a characteristic tear drop shaped appearance. What is the most likely diagnosis?

A. Fibroadenoma
B. Duct papilloma
C. Phylloides tumour
D. Duct carcinoma
E. Paget's disease

Extended matching questions

Theme: **Management of breast cancer**

A. Cyclophosphamide
B. Trastuzumab (Herceptin)
C. Tamoxifen
D. Anastrozole
E. Doxorubicin
F. Raloxifene
G. Vincristine
H. Dexamethasone
I. Paclitaxel
J. Faslodex

For each scenario described below, choose the single most appropriate answer from the above list of options. Each option may be used once, more than once or not at all.

1. A therapeutic agent highly recommended in the treatment of lymph-node-positive Her 2-positive breast cancer. ☐

2. A selective oestrogen receptor modulator drug useful in the treatment of breast cancer but associated with risks of endometrial cancer and pulmonary embolism. ☐

3. An aromatase inhibitor useful in the treatment of early breast cancer in post-menopausal women. ☐

4. A therapeutic agent useful in the treatment of breast cancer but known to cause left ventricular failure and pulmonary toxicity. ☐

5. A therapeutic agent useful in the treatment of breast cancer but known to cause bladder cancer. ☐

Single best answer

1. A 14-year-old boy presents to accident and emergency complaining of sudden onset pain in his right limb. On examination you note his right limb is red, tender and notably swollen. In addition you observe he is unwilling to move his limb. Routine blood investigations reveal a white cell count of 23×10^9/l and C Reactive protein (CRP) of 98 mg/l. What is the most common aetiological cause for this presentation?

   A. *Streptococcus pyogenes*
   B. *Haemophilus influenzae*
   C. *Salmonella*
   D. *Staphylococcus aureus*
   E. *Brucella*

2. An 8-year-old boy presents with a painful left limb. On examination you note he is pyrexic with a temperature of 38.2°C. You suspect a diagnosis of acute osteomyelitis. Which investigation is most likely to lead to a diagnosis?

   A. MRI of the affected limb
   B. Plain limb X-ray
   C. Erythrocyte sedimentation rate (ESR)
   D. White cell count
   E. C-reactive protein (CRP)

3. A 69-year-old man with Paget's disease presents with a painful right leg. He comments it is particularly painful when walking. A plain limb X-ray reveals evidence of bone destruction and a 'sunray' like appearance of his right femur. What is the most likely diagnosis?

   A. Osteoid osteoma
   B. Chondroma

   C. Ewing's sarcoma
   D. Osteoclastoma
   E. Osteosarcoma

4. A man presents to his GP with a painful right shoulder made worse by movement. On examination you note his pain is exacerbated by lifting his arm above his head or across his body. What is the most likely diagnosis?

   A. Subacromial impingement
   B. Acromioclavicular osteoarthritis
   C. Rotator cuff tear
   D. Calcific tendinitis
   E. Frozen shoulder

5. A woman presents to her GP with a painful right shoulder. On examination you note that her pain is made worse on abduction. What is the most likely diagnosis?

   A. Subacromial impingement
   B. Acromioclavicular osteoarthritis
   C. Rotator cuff tear
   D. Calcific tendinitis
   E. Frozen shoulder

6. A rugby player presents to his GP complaining of a painful left shoulder following a local match. On examination you note reduced active but full passive movement. In addition you note evidence of muscle wasting and tenderness on palpation. What is the most likely diagnosis?

   A. Subacromial impingement
   B. Acromioclavicular osteoarthritis

Extended matching questions

Theme: **Fractures**

- **A.** Clavicle
- **B.** Humeral neck
- **C.** Humeral shaft
- **D.** Scaphoid
- **E.** Distal radius
- **F.** Pelvis
- **G.** Femoral shaft
- **H.** Intracapsular neck of femur
- **I.** Tibial
- **J.** Scapula

For each scenario described below, choose the single most appropriate answer from the above list of options. Each option may be used once, more than once or not at all.

1. Commonly seen in osteoporotic postmenopausal ladies who fall on an outstretched hand. ☐

2. Occurs as a result of falling on an outstretched arm. May be associated with radial nerve injury. ☐

3. Associated with external rotation and adduction of the leg. ☐

4. Swelling and pain on wrist movement. Notably difficult to diagnose on an X-ray. ☐

5. Associated with damage to the medial femoral circumflex artery. ☐

Theme: **Fracture complications**

- **A.** Crush syndrome
- **B.** Compartment syndrome
- **C.** Algodystrophy
- **D.** Non-union
- **E.** Malunion
- **F.** Contracture
- **G.** Compensation neurosis
- **H.** Fat embolus
- **I.** Pneumonia
- **J.** Renal stone

For each scenario described below, choose the single most appropriate answer from the above list of options. Each option may be used once, more than once or not at all.

1. An elderly woman complaining of a productive cough and shortness of breath following a hip fracture. ☐

2. Occurs typically on day 3 after the fracture is sustained. Associated features include confusion, dyspnoea and hypoxia. ☐

3. Failing of fracture healing within the expected time period. Typically seen with scaphoid fractures. ☐

4. A serious condition associated with increased tissue pressure, vascular occlusion and soft tissue necrosis. ☐

5. A condition whereby a fracture unites in a non anatomical position and is associated with poor fracture healing. ☐

Single best answer

1. A 35-year-old man presents with a lump between his thyroid notch and hyoid bone which moves upwards on tongue protrusion. What is the most likely diagnosis?

   A. Lymphoma
   B. Thyroglossal cyst
   C. Branchial cyst
   D. Carotid body tumour
   E. Carcinoma

2. An 18-year-old woman presents with a cyst in the upper anterior border of her sternocleidomastoid muscle. What is the most likely diagnosis?

   A. Lymphoma
   B. Thyroglossal cyst
   C. Branchial cyst
   D. Carotid body tumour
   E. Carcinoma

3. A middle aged man presents with a lump in his neck. On examination you note it is oval shaped, non tender and pulsatile in nature. What is the most likely diagnosis?

   A. Lymphoma
   B. Thyroglossal cyst
   C. Branchial cyst
   D. Carotid body tumour
   E. Carcinoma

4. A 76-year-old man complains of swollen neck glands. On examination you note swelling and tenderness of both his parotid glands and the presence of purulent saliva on gentle palpation of his parotids. What is the most likely diagnosis?

   A. Lymphoma
   B. Pleomorphic adenoma
   C. Parotitis
   D. Parotid calculi
   E. Adenolymphoma (Warthin's tumour)

5. A 65-year-old man presents with a painless mass in his right parotid gland. He comments he has noticed the mass grow slowly over time. What is the most likely diagnosis?

   A. Lymphoma
   B. Pleomorphic adenoma
   C. Parotitis
   D. Parotid calculi
   E. Adenolymphoma (Warthin's tumour)

6. A 67-year-old woman presents with a painless mass in her left parotid gland. She comments she has noticed the mass grow slowly over time but did not feel it was anything to worry about as it was not painful in nature. What is the most likely diagnosis?

   A. Lymphoma
   B. Pleomorphic adenoma
   C. Parotitis
   D. Parotid calculi
   E. Adenolymphoma (Warthin's tumour)

7. An 18-year-old man presents to his GP with difficulty in swallowing. On examination you note swelling and tenderness of his tonsils. He is anxious as he does not want surgery. The following are all indications for a tonsillectomy EXCEPT?

   A. Sore throats being due to tonsillitis
   B. Five or more episodes of sore throat per year

Single best answer

1. A 25-year-old man is admitted to accident and emergency following a motorbike accident. You are asked to perform a primary survey and begin to assess his airway. The following are all conditions that are easily detected or excluded in a primary survey EXCEPT?

   A. Airway obstruction
   B. Tension pneumothorax
   C. Flail chest
   D. Cardiac tamponade
   E. Myocardial infarction

2. A 32-year-old man is rushed to hospital following a head on collision with a heavy goods vehicle. On examination his GCS score is 5/15. His oxygen saturation is 95% on 15 litres of oxygen, his blood pressure is 109/55 mmHg and his pulse rate is 132 beats/min. Having completed the primary survey you instruct the nurse to insert a urinary catheter. The nurse is hesitant to do so because she is concerned about urethral damage. The following are all suggestive of urethral damage EXCEPT?

   A. Blood at the urethral meatus
   B. Low riding prostate
   C. Scrotal bruising
   D. Perineal bruising
   E. Pelvic fracture

3. A 45-year-old man is admitted to accident and emergency having fallen from his horse while fox hunting. His blood pressure is 95/40 mmHg and pulse rate 124 beats/min. You note he is bleeding heavily from his right leg and shoulder. You diagnose grade III haemorrhagic shock and begin to aggressively fluid resuscitate. The following are all features of type III haemorrhagic shock EXCEPT?

   A. Narrowed pulse pressure
   B. Respiratory rate of 30–40 breaths/min
   C. Oliguria
   D. Confusion
   E. Blood loss of 750–1500 ml

4. A 32-year-old man presents to accident and emergency following a stabbing to his left chest. On examination he is severely breathless with a respiratory rate of 30 breaths/min. There is right sided deviation of his trachea with hyper-resonance on percussion and absent breath sounds on the left side. You insert a large bore intravenous cannula through the 2nd intercostal space midclavicular line. What is the most likely diagnosis?

   A. Tension pneumothorax
   B. Open pneumothorax
   C. Massive haemothorax
   D. Flail chest
   E. Cardiac tamponade

5. A 55-year-old man presents to accident and emergency following a stabbing to his chest. On examination you note an open wound on the right side of his chest. The patient is severely breathless. His oxygen saturation is 85% on room air. You apply an occlusive dressing to his wound, taping three of the four sides to the skin. His oxygen saturation begins to improve. What is the most likely diagnosis?

   A. Tension pneumothorax
   B. Open pneumothorax

C. Massive haemothorax

D. Flail chest

E. Cardiac tamponade

6. A 32-year-old woman is admitted to accident and emergency following a stabbing to her left chest. On examination she is notably breathless. Her left chest is dull to percussion and breath sounds are absent. What is the most likely diagnosis?

A. Tension pneumothorax

B. Open pneumothorax

C. Massive haemothorax

D. Flail chest

E. Cardiac tamponade

7. A 52-year-old building contractor is brought to accident and emergency having fallen from a height onto his chest. He is notably breathless and in severe pain. On examination you note crepitus on chest palpation and paradoxical movement of the lower segment of his right chest. What is the most likely diagnosis?

A. Tension pneumothorax

B. Open pneumothorax

C. Massive haemothorax

D. Flail chest

E. Cardiac tamponade

8. A 15-year-old boy is rushed to accident and emergency following a stab injury to the chest. On examination his blood pressure is 95/45 mmHg and pulse rate is 132 beats/min. You note that his heart sounds are muffled and suspect a diagnosis of cardiac tamponade. The following are all features of cardiac tamponade EXCEPT?

A. Increased venous pressure on inspiration

B. Increased systolic pressure on inspiration

C. Tachycardia

D. Distended neck veins

E. Hypotension

9. A 23-year-old boxer is admitted to accident and emergency following a blow to his head. On examination he localises to pain and opens his eyes to pain. His speech is notably confused. The following are all useful in the assessment of patients with a head injury EXCEPT?

A. Response to pain

B. Response to voice

C. Severity of headache

D. Alertness

E. Motor function

10. A 45-year-old boxer is brought to accident and emergency following a blow to his head which left him unconscious. In the department he regains consciousness but later deteriorates dramatically. An urgent CT head scan is ordered which confirms the diagnosis. What is the most likely diagnosis?

A. Extradural haematoma

B. Subdural haematoma

C. Contusion

D. Intracerebral haemorrhage

E. Axonal injury

11. A 75-year-old chronic alcoholic presents to accident and emergency following a fall. On examination she appears drowsy and her GCS drops from 12 to 8. You order an urgent CT head scan. What is the most likely diagnosis?

A. Extradural haematoma

B. Subdural haematoma

C. Contusion

D. Intracerebral haemorrhage

E. Axonal injury

12. A 23-year-old woman presents to accident and emergency following being stabbed in the back with a knife. On examination you note weakness in her right limb and loss of proprioception below the level of the injury site. You also note loss of temperature and pain on the opposite side below the site of injury. What is the most likely diagnosis?

A. Central cord syndrome
B. Posterior cord syndrome
C. Anterior cord syndrome
D. Brown Sequard syndrome
E. Spinal shock

13. A 32-year-old woman is admitted to accident and emergency following an incident with a chip pan. On examination you note evidence of erythema and blistering to her hands and face. Her blood pressure is 95/66 mmHg and pulse rate 120 beats/min. You decide to commence urgent fluid resuscitation. What is the most ideal size of cannula that you would aim to insert in this situation?

A. 14G
B. 16G
C. 18G
D. 20G
E. 22G

14. A 5-year-old boy is admitted to accident and emergency following contact with a hot pan. On examination you note erythema and mottling of his right hand. His blood pressure is 100/60 mmHg and pulse rate 65 beats/min. You decide to initiate fluid resuscitation but find it difficult to obtain good access in both his arms. You fast bleep the registrar and while waiting note his blood pressure is quickly dropping. What is the next most appropriate step in management bearing in mind the child's age?

A. Central line
B. Venous cut down
C. Femoral line
D. Arterial line
E. Intraosseous needle in the proximal tibia

Extended matching questions

Theme: Glasgow coma scale

A. 6
B. 7
C. 8
D. 9
E. 10
F. 11
G. 12
H. 13
I. 14
J. 15

For each scenario described below, choose the single most appropriate answer from the above list of options. Each option may be used once, more than once or not at all.

1. Obeys commands, with normal speech and spontaneous eye movement. ☐

2. Flexes to pain, with incomprehensible sounds and no eye movement. ☐

3. Withdraws to pain with confused speech and eyes that open to pain. ☐

4. No motor response with normal speech and spontaneous eye movement. ☐

5. Inappropriate speech associated with obeying commands and eyes opening on command. ☐

Single best answer

1. A 62-year-old man presents with sudden onset loin pain, urinary frequency and dysuria. On examination he is pyrexic with a temperature of 38.2°C. He appears notably confused. What is the next most appropriate initial investigation?

   A. Urinalysis and culture
   B. Abdominal ultrasound
   C. Intravenous urogram
   D. Abdominal X-ray
   E. Prostate specific antigen

2. A 23-year-old woman presents with urinary frequency and dysuria. Routine observations confirm a temperature of 38.7°C. Blood cultures are taken which demonstrate the growth of gram negative organisms. Which management plan would you instigate first?

   A. Oral antibiotics
   B. Intravenous antibiotics
   C. Oral fluids
   D. Urinary catheterisation
   E. Analgesia

3. A 45-year-old man presents with urinary frequency, dysuria and haematuria. On examination you note suprapubic tenderness. What is the most likely diagnosis?

   A. Pyelonephritis
   B. Interstitial cystitis
   C. Prostatitis
   D. Acute cystitis
   E. Epididymo-orchitis

4. A 41-year-old man presents with urinary frequency, dysuria and urgency. Urine cultures are taken which reveal no bacterial organisms. What is the most likely diagnosis?

   A. Pyelonephritis
   B. Interstitial cystitis
   C. Prostatitis
   D. Acute cystitis
   E. Epididymo-orchitis

5. A 62-year-old man presents with urinary frequency and dysuria. On examination you note tenderness in the lower abdomen. On rectal examination you note tenderness on palpation of his prostate. What is the most likely diagnosis?

   A. Pyelonephritis
   B. Interstitial cystitis
   C. Prostatitis
   D. Acute cystitis
   E. Epididymo-orchitis

6. A 25-year-old sexually active man presents with testicular pain and vomiting. On examination you note his testicles are swollen and tender. A urine dipstick reveals 3+ leucocytes, 2+ nitrites but no blood. What is the most likely diagnosis?

   A. Pyelonephritis
   B. Interstitial cystitis
   C. Prostatitis
   D. Acute cystitis
   E. Epididymo-orchitis

7. A 57-year-old man presents with loin pain and haematuria. On examination you note a mass in his right loin. You suspect the diagnosis of renal cancer. The following are all features of renal cell carcinoma EXCEPT?

   A. Polycythaemia
   B. Raised alkaline phosphatase
   C. Raised erythrocyte sedimentation rate (ESR)
   D. Hypocalcaemia
   E. Hypertension

8. A 49-year-old woman presents with loin pain and haematuria. On examination you note a mass in her right loin. Which investigation is most likely to lead to a diagnosis?

   A. Urea and electrolytes
   B. Abdominal CT scan
   C. Chest X-ray
   D. Intravenous urogram
   E. Urinalysis

9. A middle aged man is recently diagnosed with renal cell carcinoma of his left kidney without evidence of distant metastasis. What is the next most appropriate step in management?

   A. Embolisation of the renal artery
   B. Radiotherapy
   C. Chemotherapy
   D. Radical nephrectomy
   E. Hormonal treatments

10. A 26-year-old man presents with severe colicky pain in his right loin which radiates to his right groin. A urine dipstick is positive for blood. An intravenous urogram is requested which demonstrates a ureteric stone approximately 3 mm in size. Following appropriate analgesia, which management plan is most appropriate in the first instance?

    A. Extracorporeal shockwave lithotripsy
    B. Percutaneous nephrolithotomy
    C. Open surgical removal
    D. Ureteric stenting
    E. Allow for the stone to pass spontaneously

11. A 26-year-old man presents with severe colicky pain in his right loin which radiates to his right groin. A urine dipstick proves positive for blood and nitrites. An intravenous urogram is requested which demonstrates a ureteric stone approximately 4 mm in size. Which management plan would you instigate first?

    A. Analgesia
    B. Commence an alpha blocker
    C. Open surgical removal
    D. Arrange referral for extracorporeal shockwave lithotripsy
    E. Antibiotics

12. A 65-year-old smoker presents with painless haematuria. Routine examination proves unremarkable. Routine blood investigations reveal a urea of 15.4 mmol/l and creatinine of 154 micromol/l. You suspect a diagnosis of bladder cancer. What is the next most appropriate initial investigation?

    A. Cystoscopy and biospy
    B. Chest X-ray
    C. Intravenous urogram
    D. Abdominal MRI scan
    E. Abdominal CT scan

13. A 60-year-old man presents with painless haematuria. A cystoscopy confirms the presence of a tumour in his bladder, which is malignant on biopsy. He undergoes a staging CT scan which confirms involvement of the superficial muscle and no evidence of distant metastases. What is the next most appropriate step in management?

    A. Radical cystectomy
    B. Radiotherapy
    C. Systemic chemotherapy
    D. Transurethral resection
    E. Watchful waiting

14. A 72-year-old man presents with urinary frequency and nocturia. You suspect a diagnosis of benign prostatic hyperplasia. According to the International Prostate Symptom Score his

symptoms are classified as mild. What is the next most appropriate step in management?

A. Watchful waiting
B. Radical prostatectomy
C. Radiotherapy
D. 5 alpha reductase inhibitors
E. Alpha blockers

15. A mother brings her 1-year-old son for a routine check up with his GP. On examination the GP notes failure of testicular descent into the scrotum. The child is referred for surgery. The following are all complications of undescended testes EXCEPT?

A. Infertility
B. Femoral hernia
C. Torsion
D. Inguinal hernia
E. Testicular carcinoma

16. A 36-year-old man presents with a painless lump in his scrotum. On examination you note a non tender hard lump in his testis. What is the next most appropriate initial investigation to help establish a diagnosis?

A. Abdominal CT scan
B. Chest CT scan
C. Serum alpha fetoprotein
D. Serum lactate dehydrogenase
E. Serum beta HCG

17. A 35-year-old man presents with a lump in his scrotum. On examination the lump is translucent and non tender. You find it difficult to identify the testes and epididymis separately. What is the most likely diagnosis?

A. Hydrocele
B. Epididymo-orchitis
C. Epididymal cyst
D. Testicular tumour
E. Testicular torsion

18. A 24-year-old man presents with a lump in his scrotum. On examination the lump is non-translucent and extremely tender. You find it difficult to identify the testes and epididymis. What is the most likely diagnosis?

A. Hydrocele
B. Epididymo-orchitis
C. Epididymal cyst
D. Testicular tumour
E. Testicular torsion

19. A 32-year-old man presents with a lump in his scrotum. On examination the lump is translucent, separate from the testes and is non tender. What is the most likely diagnosis?

A. Hydrocele
B. Epididymo-orchitis
C. Epididymal cyst
D. Testicular tumour
E. Testicular torsion

20. A 16-year-old boy presents with sudden onset severe pain in his left scrotum and vomiting. On examination you note evidence of scrotal erythema and tenderness on palpation. A urine dipstick proves negative. What is the most likely diagnosis?

A. Epididymitis
B. Hydrocele
C. Orchitis
D. Appendicitis
E. Testicular torsion

Extended matching questions

Theme: Investigations

A. Urine dipstick

B. Cystoscopy

C. Serum prostate specific antigen

D. Renal ultrasound scan

E. Abdominal CT scan

F. Serum urea and creatinine

G. Urodynamic studies (cystometrogram)

H. Abdominal X-ray of kidneys, ureters and bladder (KUB)

I. Intravenous urography

J. Renal aortography

For each scenario described below, choose the single most appropriate answer from the above list of options. Each option may be used once, more than once or not at all.

1. A patient presenting with dysuria and frequency. Routine observations reveal a temperature of 38.6°C.

2. A 25-year-old long-distance runner presenting with severe right-sided loin pain and vomiting.

3. A middle aged man presenting with urinary hesitancy, a poor stream and terminal dribbling post micturition with evidence of renal dysfunction.

4. A 75-year-old man presenting with urinary frequency, nocturia and weight loss. An irregular mass is evident on the prostate on digital examination.

5. A middle aged female who has had 5 vaginal deliveries presenting with urinary leakage when coughing or laughing.

Single best questions

1. A 35-year-old man is 2 days post-repair of an inguinal hernia. He complains of increasing shortness of breath. Routine observations reveal an oxygen saturation of 74% on room air. On chest examination you note course crepitations bi-basally. You perform an arterial blood gas which demonstrates a PO_2 of 7.4 kPa and PCO_2 of 8.2 kPa. You suspect the possibility of respiratory failure. The following are all true statements regarding respiratory failure EXCEPT?

   A. Type I respiratory failure is associated with a low PCO_2

   B. Type II respiratory failure is associated with a low PO_2

   C. Respiratory failure is associated with a respiratory rate of greater than 30 breaths/min

   D. Respiratory failure is associated with a PCO_2 of greater than 7 kPa.

   E. Type I respiratory failure is due to inadequate ventilation

2. A 65-year-old obese man is 3 days post anterior resection for rectal cancer. During the ward round he becomes notably short of breath and appears confused. Routine observations reveal an oxygen saturation of 85% on room air. You are concerned he has developed respiratory failure due to a pulmonary embolus. The following are all causes of respiratory failure EXCEPT?

   A. Airway obstruction

   B. Asthma

   C. Anaemia

   D. Low serum magnesium

   E. Low serum phosphate

3. A 54-year-old woman is 2 days post an open appendicectomy for perforated appendicitis. She is reviewed on the ward round and comments she is still experiencing abdominal soreness. On examination she is notably tender over the lower abdomen. The nurses inform you that she has a temperature of 38.9°C, a blood pressure of 100/54 mmHg and pulse rate of 75 beats/min. Her blood results reveal a white cell count of 21×10^9/l and C Reactive protein (CRP) of 154 mg/l. What is the most likely diagnosis?

   A. Cardiogenic shock

   B. Hypovolaemic shock

   C. Septic shock

   D. Obstructive shock

   E. Anaphylactic shock

4. A 55-year-old woman with severe intermittent claudication is admitted for an elective arteriogram and possible angioplasty of her right leg. She has a past medical history of rheumatoid arthritis and mildly impaired renal function. Current medication includes penicillamine. Admission blood investigations reveal a urea of 12.8 mmol/l and creatinine of 163 micromol/l with previous results being in a similar range. However, following the arteriogram her urea and creatinine have increased to 32.8 mmol/l and 363 micromol/l respectively. What is the most likely cause of her acute renal failure?

   A. Age

   B. Minimal fluid intake

   C. Radiological contrast nephropathy

   D. Penicillamine

   E. Past medical history of renal failure

5. You are a house officer in breast surgery and are clerking in a 45-year-old woman who is being admitted for excision of a benign breast lump. She has no known past medical or surgical history. Which investigation is most highly recommended prior to her surgery?

   A. Full blood count
   B. ECG
   C. Chest X-ray
   D. Urea and electrolytes
   E. None of the above

6. You are a house officer in general surgery and are clerking in a 65-year-old man who is being admitted electively for an inguinal hernia repair. His past medical history includes chronic obstructive pulmonary disease (COPD). He states he has had a chest X-ray over 6 weeks ago. Which investigation is most highly recommended prior to his surgery?

   A. Full blood count
   B. ECG
   C. Chest X-ray
   D. Urea and electrolytes
   E. Clotting screen

7. You are a house officer in surgery assessing a 69-year-old man planned for a thyroidectomy for a known history of hyperthyroidism the following week. He has no other past medical or surgical history. The following investigations are all recommended prior to his surgery EXCEPT?

   A. ECG
   B. Full blood count
   C. Urea and electrolytes
   D. Clotting screen
   E. Thyroid function tests

8. You are a house officer in colorectal surgery and are clerking in a 68-year-old man who is planned for an anterior resection the following week. His past medical history includes ischaemic heart disease but no history of a myocardial infarction. The following investigations are all recommended prior to his surgery EXCEPT?

   A. Chest X-ray
   B. ECG
   C. Full blood count
   D. Urea and electrolytes
   E. Lung function tests

9. You are clerking a 63-year-old man planned for an anterior resection for rectal cancer the following week. His past medical history includes diabetes, ischaemic heart disease and atrial fibrillation. His current medication includes metformin, aspirin and warfarin. The following are all important steps to take prior to his surgery EXCEPT?

   A. Phosphate enema on the day of surgery
   B. TED stockings and enoxaparin injections while an inpatient
   C. Stopping aspirin at least 7 days before his surgery
   D. Stopping warfarin at least 3 days before his surgery
   E. Use of an insulin sliding scale prior to his surgery

10. A 32-year-old man is complaining of increasing pain 2 days post inguinal hernia repair. He is currently prescribed paracetamol 1 g four times a day. What is the next most appropriate step in management?

    A. Codeine
    B. Tramadol
    C. Morphine
    D. Co codamol
    E. Diclofenac

Single best answer

1. A 23-year-old woman with ulcerative colitis undergoes a subtotal colectomy and ileostomy formation following failure of medical treatment for fulminant colitis. The following are all complications of ileostomy formation EXCEPT?

   A. Hernia
   B. Prolapse
   C. Electrolyte imbalance
   D. Parastomal dermatitis
   E. Intrahepatic calculi

2. An elderly man presents with left sided abdominal pain and dark red rectal bleeding. Past medical history includes ischaemic heart disease. He is known to smoke 40 cigarettes per day over a 30-year period. On examination you note obvious distension of his abdomen. Routine observations demonstrate a blood pressure of 105/65 mmHg and pulse rate of 130 beats/minute. He is apyrexial. What is the most likely diagnosis?

   A. Lymphocytic colitis
   B. Ulcerative colitis
   C. Ischaemic colitis
   D. Diverticulitis
   E. Microscopic colitis

3. A 65-year-old man presents with sudden onset abdominal pain. On further questioning he comments he has not opened his bowels for 3 days and has been vomiting intermittently. On examination his abdomen is grossly distended and he is notably tender throughout. A plain radiograph of his abdomen demonstrates evidence of sigmoid volvulus. What is the next most appropriate step in management to achieve definitive resolution?

   A. Emergency laparotomy
   B. Flexible sigmoidoscopic decompression with a flatus tube
   C. Intravenous fluids
   D. Nasogastric tube insertion
   E. Intravenous fluids and insertion of a nasogastric tube

4. A 65-year-old man presents with rectal bleeding and weight loss. You advise him for the need of a colonoscopy which he refuses. You arrange an abdominal CT scan which demonstrates evidence of a right sided colonic tumour mass. The following are all possible features of right sided colonic tumours EXCEPT?

   A. Weight loss
   B. Abdominal pain
   C. Iron deficiency anaemia
   D. Vitamin B12 deficiency anaemia
   E. Hepatomegaly

5. A middle aged woman presents with bleeding when opening her bowels. She comments the blood is bright red in nature and can be seen on the toilet paper and in the pan following defecation. A proctoscopy is performed which helps confirm the diagnosis. Which management plan would you suggest first?

   A. Review in 2 months
   B. Barron banding
   C. Surgery
   D. Cryotherapy
   E. Injection sclerotherapy

6. A 55-year-old man presents to his GP complaining of perianal discomfort. On examination you note a discrete swelling in

Answers Rheumatology

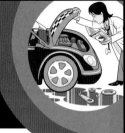

Single best answer

1 B. Osteoarthritis commonly affects the distal interphalangeal joints and first carpometacarpal joints of the hands. The first metatarsophalangeal joint of the foot is also commonly affected.

2 D. The likely diagnosis is osteoarthritis and the most useful investigation is an X-ray of the knee. It may demonstrate narrowing of the joint space, presence of osteophytes, cyst formation or joint erosion.

3 E. A classic description of osteoarthritis. Paracetamol is the simplest and safest painkiller and the best one to try first. However, NSAIDs, which have more side effects, may often be necessary. Heat and hydrotherapy may be used in conjunction with painkillers. Surgery and steroids would only be considered if these modalities failed to control symptoms.

4 C. A classic description of rheumatoid arthritis. Rheumatoid factor is usually positive in 60–70% of cases.

5 A. The diagnosis is rheumatoid arthritis. Anaemia is a common manifestation of the condition. In addition patients may suffer from lymphadenopathy, carpal tunnel syndrome and secondary Sjögren's syndrome.

6 E. Methotrexate is a disease-modifying drug (DMARD) which helps to prevent irreversible joint damage with ongoing symptoms. NSAIDs and COX 2 inhibitors have no disease-modifying effect and are used as single agents only in the early stages. TNF alpha blockers are not first-line treatment and surgery is confined to certain situations.

7 A. A classic description of ankylosing spondylitis. Other features include iritis, aortic incompetence and lung fibrosis.

8 C. Reactive arthritis consists of a triad of three symptoms: arthritis, urethritis and conjunctivitis.

9 B. Psoriatic arthritis commonly affects the distal interphalangeal joints on a background of psoriasis, particularly in those with nail disease.

10 E. The gram positive coccus is *Staphylococcus aureus*, most appropriately treated with intravenous flucloxacillin and oral fucidin.

11 B. The patient is probably suffering from systemic lupus erythematosus. Antinuclear antibodies are positive in most cases.

12 C. The woman is suffering from systemic sclerosis which is primarily a clinical diagnosis. Anti centromere antibodies are diagnostic.

13 A. Dermatomyositis commonly presents with a purple peri orbital skin rash. Other features include erythematous plaques over the fingers and knuckles.

14 E. Muscle biopsy is the definitive test for polymyositis.

15 A. The diagnosis is Sjögren's syndrome. Anti-Ro and Anti-La antibodies are present in 60–70% of patients.

16 B. Henoch–Schönlein purpura commonly presents as a purpuric rash on the legs and buttocks. Other features include abdominal pain, arthritis and haematuria.

17 D. This man has gout. NSAIDs are the treatment of choice.

18 D. This woman has pseudogout secondary to haemachromatosis. Joint fluid microscopy would demonstrate brick shaped crystals which would be positively birefringent under polarized light.

19 D. A classic description of osteomalacia.

20 D. Bisphosphonates are the first-line treatment in osteoporosis but reducing alcohol intake and stopping smoking are also advised.

21 B. Alkaline phosphatase may be as high as 1000 U/l.

Extended matching questions

Theme: Arthritis

1 F. Additional features include involvement of the first metatarsophalangeal joint of the foot and bony swellings at the distal interphalangeal joints (Heberden's nodes).

2 H. Additional features include ulnar deviation, hyperextension of the proximal interphalangeal joint (swan neck deformity) and flexion of the proximal interphalangeal joint (Boutonniere deformity).

3 G. Classic presentation of psoriatic arthritis. There is an increased frequency of ankylosing spondylitis in such patients.

4 E. Classic presentation of reactive arthritis. Treatment involves the use of NSAIDs, corticosteroids and antibiotics.

5 A. Ankylosing spondylitis may be an additional feature.

Theme: Connective tissue disease

1 C. Additional features include arthritis, cranial nerve abnormalities and pleural effusions.

2 D. Classic description of discoid lupus.

3 A. Additional features include an increased risk of deep vein thrombosis, stroke and myocardial infarction.

4 F. Additional skin changes may include a photosensitive rash on the face and erythematous plaques on the fingers.

5 B. Additional features include lung fibrosis, myocardial fibrosis, renal failure, joint deformities and Raynaud's phenomenon.

Theme: Vasculitis

1 A. A classic presentation of polymyalgia most appropriately managed with steroids.

2 B. Temporal arteritis is associated with an increased risk of stroke.

3 H. Additional features may include mononeuritis multiplex, hypertension and weight loss.

There is a strong link with hepatitis B antigen with regards to pathogenesis.

4 J. Classic presentation of microscopic polyangiitis. Management typically involves prednisolone and cyclophosphamide.

5 I. Typical presentation of Behçet's disease. The red coloured lumps are indicative of erythema nodosum.

Theme: Drugs

1 B. Additional side effects include muscle weakness, double vision and a yellow discoloration of the skin.

2 E. Hydroxychloroquine is specifically associated with retinopathy.

3 F. A well recognised side effect of auranofin.

4 D. Additional side effects include blood dyscrasias, gastrointestinal disturbances and central nervous system reactions.

5 G. Additional side effects include thrombocytopenia and hepatoxicity.

Theme: Back pain

1 G. Additional features may include sacral numbness and impotence.

2 C. This is most appropriately investigated by CT or MRI scans with surgical decompression being the mainstay form of treatment.

3 A. Treatment typically involves bed rest, analgesia and physiotherapy.

4 B. This is commonly due to the slipping of one vertebra on another, most commonly L4/L5.

5 D. Additional features include loss of lumbar lordosis, kyphosis and reduced chest expansion.

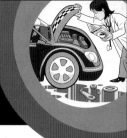

Single best answer

1 D. This patient is most likely to be suffering from COPD due to his long-standing smoking history.

2 C. An arterial blood gas is necessary. It will determine the patient's oxygen saturation and whether the patient is retaining carbon dioxide. As a result oxygen therapy can be tailored accordingly.

3 B. Individuals with COPD typically depend on a degree of hypoxia to maintain respiratory drive so it is best to commence low oxygen concentrations via a venturi mask. The oxygen saturation and arterial blood gas results should be regularly assessed to determine correct oxygen therapy.

4 D. The diagnosis is obstructive sleep apnoea. All of the listed options can occur in obstructive sleep apnoea but daytime sleepiness is the most common.

5 A. A typical presentation of cystic fibrosis. The presence of clubbing suggests a chronic respiratory disease process as opposed to an acute infection.

6 E. High-resolution chest CT is the investigation of choice.

7 D. Individuals with cystic fibrosis are at risk of respiratory infection. Antibiotics are therefore of paramount importance in those with exacerbation of symptoms.

8 D. A sodium value above 60 mmol/l is diagnostic.

9 C. Animal handling as a vet is likely to be the explanation in this case.

10 B. The diagnosis of asthma depends on a compatible history in combination with demonstration of variable expiratory airflow limitation. There is no single test that is appropriate for everyone. It is the variability of PEFR that is the key to diagnosis. A reduced PEFR is seen in COPD so it is the variability that is important.

11 B. A peak flow of less than 80% of the predicted value is best treated with a low dose inhaled steroid.

12 A. Nebulised salbutamol or terbutaline in addition to oral steroids are the initial treatment of acute severe asthma. Oral steroids are as effective as intravenous steroids.

13 A. *Streptococcus pneumoniae* is the most common cause of community acquired pneumonia where a pathogen is isolated.

14 C. The mortality associated with community acquired pneumonia is dependent on the CURB 65 score as recommended by the British Thoracic Society. A respiratory rate of 30 breaths per minute is a key risk factor.

15 D. *Mycoplasma pneumoniae* is known to cause erythema multiforme and haemolytic anaemia.

16 A. This type of pneumonia is often seen following contact with infected birds such as parrots.

17 C. *Staphylococcus aureus* pneumonia is often seen in intravenous drug abusers.

18 E. Legionellosis is linked to contamination of water systems in hotels and hospitals. Additional features include diarrhoea and confusion.

19 A. For mild cases of pneumonia oral amoxicillin 500 mg 8 hourly for 7 days is the usual starting regimen.

20 D. Chest X-ray is the gold standard investigation in pneumonia.

21 D. *Mycobacterium tuberculosis* is often seen in Asian immigrants and can result in haemoptysis.

22 B. Macrophages are responsible for engulfing the bacilli.

23 B. Sputum staining with Ziehl–Neelsen stain for acid- and alcohol-fast bacilli or an auramine–phenol fluorescent test would be the next appropriate investigation.

24 C. Streptomycin is rarely used and is reserved for cases of isoniazid resistance.

25 A. Rifampicin causes pink coloured urine.

26 E. This patient has a diagnosis of sarcoidosis. Skin and ocular disturbances are the most common extrapulmonary features of the condition.

27 E. However, if there were no peripheral lesions to biopsy, a transbronchial biopsy may be necessary.

28 C. A classic description of cryptogenic fibrosing alveolitis. The presence of clubbing makes this more likely than the other possibilities.

29 A. World-wide, there are differences, but forking mouldy hay (farmer's lung) is the most common cause from the listed options.

30 D. Evidence of bilateral diffuse pleural thickening would allow a benefit claim to be pursued.

31 A. Smoking is the most common cause of lung cancer.

32 C. Adenocarcinomas are the most common lung cancers in non smokers and in those exposed to asbestos.

33 E. This patient has clinical features of Cushing's syndrome seen commonly in small cell lung cancers. This is due to production of ACTH from Kuchitsky cells.

34 A. Clubbing would be the most common extra pulmonary feature from the listed options.

35 A. Surgery is the most suitable treatment here as it is a small confined tumour. However most patients with SCLC present with advanced disease and are not suitable for surgical resection.

36 E. Protein or lactic dehydrogenase levels are important in determining whether an effusion is a transudate or exudate.

37 A. Causes of transudates include heart failure, hypoproteinaemia, hypothyroidism and Meig's syndrome to name but a few.

38 A. This patient has a pulmonary embolus best diagnosed by CTPA. CTPA is often preferred over a V Q scan as it helps to show other pathology if the diagnosis is not a confirmed pulmonary embolus.

Extended matching questions

Theme: Pneumonia

1 G. A common cause of pneumonia in cystic fibrosis or individuals who are immunocompromised.

2 E. A common cause of pneumonia in individuals with COPD.

3 B. Seen particularly in those in close contact with infected parrots. Additional features include high fever and meningism.

4 C. *Staphylococcus aureus* is a common cause of pneumonia in intravenous drug users or in patients with central venous catheters.

5 D. Likely cause of pneumonia associated with contaminated water systems in hotels.

Theme: Drugs

1 D. This drug also causes pink coloured urine and body secretions.

2 A. Ethambutol is known to result in visual disturbances such as colour blindness and central scotoma formation.

3 H. The diagnosis is *Staphylococcus aureus* pneumonia most appropriately treated with flucloxacillin.

4 B. Additional side effects include rashes and arthralgia.

5 E. This individual is at risk of aspiration pneumonia most appropriately treated with metronidazole as infection is commonly due to anaerobes.

Theme: Lung cancer

1 E. The term used to describe this finding.

2 G. Pancoast's tumour involves the brachial plexus and causes pain in the shoulder and inner arm.

3 D. Other areas of pigmentation may include the groin.

4 F. Classic features of Horner's syndrome as a result of involvement of the preganglionic sympathetic nerves.

5 A. Essentially a myasthenic syndrome associated with a defective release of acetylcholine at the neuromuscular junction.

Theme: **Diseases of the respiratory tract**

1 G. Classic definition of emphysema.

2 F. A viral infection associated with myalgia, headaches, cough and a sore throat. Management is usually symptomatic relief.

3 E. Features are essentially due to inflammatory oedema involving the larynx.

4 A. Cystic fibrosis is the most common cause of bronchiectasis.

5 H. Typical features of acute bronchitis.

Theme: **Investigative findings**

1 I. This condition is associated with a ground glass appearance progressing to a honeycomb lung on chest X-ray.

2 G. Typical X-ray features of extrinsic allergic alveolitis.

3 A. Patients with COPD have partially reversible airflow limitation with an increase in FEV_1 of less than 15% on inhalation of a β_2 agonist.

4 J. Typical presentation of pneumonia.

5 D. This is essentially a vasculitis of the upper respiratory tract, lungs and kidneys with anti neutrophil cytoplasmic antibodies found in over 90% of cases.

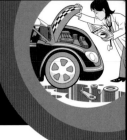
Single best answer

1 C. Pituitary tumours typically cause a bitemporal hemianopia due to compression of decussating fibres from the nasal half of each eye.

2 A. FSH and LH are usually affected first with TSH and ACTH affected last.

3 E. The commonest cause of hypopituitarism is a tumour in over 70% of cases.

4 A. Thyroid hormones and steroid hormones are essential for life and are usually given as an oral replacement dose.

5 D. Galactorrhea in a man is due to hyperprolactinaemia either due to increased secretion or decreased elimination (renal or hepatic disease). The first step in diagnosis is always to measure serum prolactin concentrations (at least three times). The neurological symptoms in this case suggest a prolactinoma and an MRI of the pituitary will then be necessary.

6 D. The diagnosis is acromegaly. The oral glucose tolerance test is the most reliable diagnostic test for this condition.

7 E. Hashimoto's thyroiditis is the most common cause of an under active thyroid.

8 B. Anaemia in individuals who are hypothyroid is typically normocytic or macrocytic.

9 D. Intravenous hydrocortisone would be the most appropriate step in management (after taking a random baseline cortisol) as he has a background history of an under active pituitary gland.

10 D. Graves' disease is the most common cause of hyperthyroidism and is the result of IgG antibodies binding to the TSH receptor.

11 E. Ophthalmoplegia is associated with Graves' disease. Additional features include exophthalmus, thyroid acropathy and pretibial myxoedema. All the other features listed in the question can occur with any cause of thyrotoxicosis.

12 D. Anti-TSH receptor antibodies are present in almost all cases of Graves' disease and are diagnostic of the disorder.

13 A. Carbimazole takes approximately 1–20 days to take effect. Propranolol will help to provide symptomatic control almost immediately.

14 A. The most common side effect is a rash but the most dangerous is agranulocytosis.

15 C. Radioactive iodine is contraindicated as it is teratogenic. Surgery is unlikely to be necessary in a pregnant patient.

16 E. The diagnosis is thyroid crisis following radioactive iodine. This is much less common now that patients are adequately prepared. As the patient is severely dehydrated intravenous fluids would be the first most appropriate step in management.

17 E. One should aim to normalize thyroid status. Hypothyroidism should be avoided as this may exacerbate visual disturbance.

18 D. Fine-needle aspiration cytology is most likely to reveal a diagnosis of malignancy.

19 D. Medullary cell thyroid cancers are associated with hypercalcaemia.

20 A. Anaplastic carcinomas are associated with a poor prognosis. Surgical resection is indicated for the few cases that are confined to the thyroid gland. There is no effective therapy for metastatic anaplastic thyroid carcinoma.

21 E. Cushing's syndrome is associated with an increased predisposition to infection and circulating lymphocytes are inhibited in the main.

22 D. The diagnosis is Addison's disease. The investigation of choice being the short tetracosactide test.

23 A. The most common cause is autoimmune in over 90% of cases.

24 C. The diagnosis here is Addisonian crisis. First-line management is intravenous hydrocortisone administered immediately after taking a blood sample for random cortisol.

25 E. The diagnosis here is secondary hypoadrenalism as a result of long-term steroid use. This is best diagnosed with a long tetracosactide test.

26 D. This woman has Cushing's syndrome. The most common cause being a pituitary adenoma.

27 D. The raised ACTH suggests the hypercortisolaemia is not of adrenal origin. Suppression of plasma cortisol following dexamethasone confirms a pituitary-dependent aetiology, typically an adenoma.

28 E. Surgical treatment is the best approach for pituitary tumours most commonly via a trans-sphenoidal approach.

29 C. The criteria for diagnosis include a low serum sodium, low plasma osmolality, a urine osmolality higher than plasma osmolality and an elevated urinary sodium.

30 E. The diagnosis here is SIADH and is treated initially with fluid restriction.

31 E. A side effect of lithium is diabetes insipidus which is diagnosed with a water deprivation test with desmopressin.

32 B. The diagnosis is hypocalcaemia. Secondary hyperparathyroidism is a physiological response to hypocalcaemia which in this case is due to a low vitamin D.

33 B. Hypercalcaemia is treated with intravenous saline as the first line management.

34 E. A diagnosis of hypocalcaemia is most commonly due to renal failure.

35 A. Plasma aldosterone to renin ratio is diagnostic for primary hyperaldosteronism showing suppressed renin and increased aldosterone.

36 D. This is a typical presentation of a phaeochromocytoma and the suspected diagnosis is confirmed by a measurement of 24-hour urinary catecholamines and metanephrines, the breakdown product of adrenaline.

37 A. This is type 2 diabetes mellitus. Of the listed options diet therapy is always the first line management, particularly in the elderly. However, metformin is usually used as well.

38 B. Metformin is particularly useful in obese individuals as it does not increase appetite.

39 E. Diarrhoea is the most common side effect. Other side effects include lactic acidosis.

40 D. This is type I diabetes mellitus and requires insulin. In view of the patient's age an intermediate-acting insulin is appropriate first-line management.

41 C. Hypoglycaemia in an unconscious patient is always treated with intravenous dextrose initially.

42 A. The diagnosis is diabetic ketoacidosis. The most urgent priority is intravenous saline closely followed by treatment with soluble insulin intravenously. Colloids are given if the patient is hypotensive.

43 C. Typical examination findings of pre-proliferative retinopathy.

44 E. Symmetrical sensory neuropathy affects the toes and soles of the feet initially. Involvement of the hands does occur which results in a stocking and glove sensory loss.

45 E. Diabetes in pregnancy can lead to neonatal hypoglycaemia due to hypersecretion of insulin from fetal islets.

46 A. The treatment of choice is always surgery.

Extended matching questions

Theme: Pituitary disease

1 D. Kallmann's syndrome is associated with gonadotrophin deficiency with absent sense of smell, colour blindness and renal impairment.

2 B. This condition is associated with pituitary infarction following postpartum haemorrhage.

3 A. Infarction or haemorrhage into a pituitary tumour. Headaches and visual loss are typical symptoms.

4 C. Typical features of the condition. The sella turcica appears devoid of pituitary tissue on radiological imaging.

5 E. Classic presentation of acromegaly which is almost always due to a pituitary tumour.

Theme: **Thyroid disease**

1 G. Inflammation of the thyroid gland due to a viral infection. Often associated with fever, neck pain and malaise.

2 E. Graves' disease is associated with the binding of IgG antibodies to the TSH receptor.

3 A. Hashimoto's thyroiditis is a common cause of thyroid under activity and is associated with goitre formation.

4 H. Likely to represent a thyroid cancer, specifically medullary cell. The increased calcium in these tumours is due to co-existing increased PTH as part of MEN-2. Hyperthyroidism can cause hypercalcaemia but not usually markedly raised levels.

5 I. A rare complication associated with deterioration of thyrotoxicosis following infection, stress or radioactive iodine.

Theme: **Diabetic complications**

1 E. Additional features include numbness, tingling and pain particularly at night.

2 C. Classic description of pre proliferative retinopathy.

3 A. Typical presentation of background retinopathy.

4 I. Additional features include diminished knee reflexes.

5 G. Symptoms are typically worse at night and are best treated with tricyclic antidepressants.

Theme: **Drugs**

1 D. Typical side effects of acarbose.

2 C. Typical side effects of metformin.

3 C. Used in obese individuals as it does not increase appetite.

4 A. A sulphonylurea which acts via closure of K^+ ATP channels leading to calcium influx and insulin release. Unlike tolbutamide, it is long acting and therefore avoided in the elderly due to the risk of hypoglycaemia.

5 F. An insulin releasing agent which helps to lower postprandial hyperglycaemia.

Theme: **Investigations**

1 B. The diagnosis is acromegaly. Glucose tolerance test is diagnostic.

2 G. Cushing's syndrome. This test will help confirm the raised cortisol.

3 J. Presentation of a phaeochromocytoma diagnosed by measurement of urinary catecholamines and their breakdown products.

4 E. Addison's disease is usually diagnosed via the short synacthen test.

5 H. This is likely to be diabetes insipidus. This is usually first investigated by measurement of urine and plasma osmolality, to look for psychogenic polydipsia, but will need a supervised water deprivation test to confirm the diagnosis.

26 C. Glomerulonephritis is the most common cause of nephrotic syndrome in Europe and the USA at this age.

27 A. Salt restriction will help to relieve the oedema.

28 C. Blood pressure control would be the first plan of action.

Extended matching questions

Theme: Renal disease

1 H. Typical presentation includes renal colic and haematuria. Diagnosis is usually made by excretion urography.

2 G. Typical features include acute loin pain, haematuria and abdominal discomfort. Individuals are at risk of developing hypertension.

3 A. The offending organism is typically β haemolytic streptococci. Additional features include hypertension and oedema of the legs and sacrum.

4 B. Management typically involves high dose prednisolone.

5 D. NSAIDs are a common cause of tubulointerstitial nephritis.

Theme: Complications of renal failure

1 D. Essentially osteosclerosis is an increase in bone density. If present in the verterbrae it can give rise to a 'rugger jersey' spine.

2 E. Congo red staining or tissue biopsy are the gold standard methods of diagnosing amyloidosis.

3 A. In this case decreased erythropoietin formation results in reduced red blood cell formation and subsequent anaemia.

4 F. This is commonly due to uraemia. Dialysis is essential in such cases.

5 B. Classic description of osteomalacia. Renal failure results in phosphate retention and impaired production of vitamin D.

Theme: Clinical features of renal disease

1 B. Classic presentation of nephrotic syndrome.

2 G. Additional features include neurological and cardiovascular abnormalities.

3 I. Patients may also experience notable weight loss and bone or chest pain due to metastases.

4 E. The patient has gout which may be associated with uric acid stone formation.

5 A. Classic presentation of nephritic syndrome.

Theme: Investigations

1 D. Renal failure may be precipitated by ACE inhibitors in patients with renal artery stenosis (presuered atheromations in this case). Magnetic resonance angiography is the gold standard for the diagnosis of renal artery stenosis.

2 E. The diagnosis is renal colic may be diagnosed by abdominal X-ray of the kidneys, ureters and bladder.

3 F. The diagnosis is urinary tract obstruction most appropriately investigated by renal ultrasound in the first instance.

4 C. This patient has a urinary tract infection. A urine dipstick together with urine microscopy and culture is essential.

5 J. This patient has stress incontinence most appropriately diagnosed by urodynamic investigations.

Theme: Management of renal disease

1 D. This patient is likely to have benign prostatic hypertrophy. Alpha blockers would help to relax the smooth muscle in the bladder neck and prostate.

2 F. The diagnosis is renal colic. Analgesia is the mainstay form of management.

3 E. This patient is likely to be suffering from a urinary tract infection and would require antibiotic therapy.

4 G. The diagnosis is nephrotic syndrome most appropriately treated with steroid therapy.

5 C. The diagnosis is renal cell carcinoma most appropriately managed by surgical intervention.

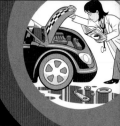

Single best answer

1 A. The diagnosis is myasthenia gravis which is initially investigated by demonstrating the presence of acetylcholine receptor antibodies. Single-fibre EMG is more sensitive for diagnosis than acetylcholine receptor antibodies but is less widely available.

2 E. The patient is demonstrating myotonia: a delay in muscle relaxation after contraction.

3 C. Typical presentation of Duchenne muscular dystrophy. Becker's usually presents later but may have similar clinical features.

4 B. Alcoholics are often at risk of thiamine (vitamin B1) deficiency which can lead to neurological abnormalities such as ataxia, nystagmus and ophthalmoplegia. Long term, there is a risk of brain damage and memory loss.

5 E. The diagnosis is Guillain–Barré syndrome which is associated with this CSF finding.

6 C. Typical presentation of median nerve damage.

7 E. Motor neurone disease is a clinical diagnosis and needs no investigative involvement. Investigations are usually performed only to rule out other neurological problems with a similar presentation.

8 B. Classic presentation of Friedreich's ataxia. Additional features include pes cavus and cardiomyopathy.

9 A. The likely diagnosis is syringomyelia which is usually investigated by spinal MRI studies.

10 C. The most likely diagnosis is spinal cord compression. From the listed options a myeloma is the most common cause of her symptoms.

11 B. This patient has spinal cord compression best managed by surgical decompression.

12 C. Typical presentation of a cluster headache. Additional features include rhinorrhoea and Horner's syndrome.

13 B. Usual features of giant cell arteritis. Visual loss is as a result of occlusion of the ciliary and central retinal artery.

14 E. The diagnosis is giant cell arteritis. High dose steroids should be the first choice of management in this case.

15 A. The diagnosis is giant cell arteritis. This condition leads to visual loss as a result of central retinal artery occlusion. As a result the retina appears white with a cherry red spot on the macula.

16 D. Typical presentation of a migraine.

17 A. The diagnosis is a migraine which is pathologically due to serotonin and nitric oxide release.

18 E. Due to his past medical history ergotamine and sumatriptan are contraindicated. The most appropriate management would be analgesia and anti-emetics. Pizotifen and methysergide are only useful if attacks are frequent in nature.

19 C. Frontal lobe tumours often lead to personality changes and apathy.

20 B. Due to distortion of normal structures at a distance from the expanding tumour a third and sixth nerve palsy are common additional findings.

21 C. Bearing in mind her age *Streptococcus pneumoniae* is most likely.

22 B. Clinical findings are suggestive of meningococcal septicaemia which requires immediate use of cefotaxime or ceftriaxone as recommended by the Meningitis Research Foundation.

23 B. Lumbar puncture is the appropriate investigation in suspected meningitis.

24 E. Most likely findings on CSF analysis in the case of bacterial meningitis.

25 E. The diagnosis is multiple sclerosis. Peripheral nerves are never affected.

26 A. The most likely diagnosis is multiple sclerosis. MRI of the brain is the investigation of choice initially.

27 E. This is due to the production of immunoglobulins to unknown antigens within the nervous system.

28 D. An autosomal dominant condition. The tremor characteristically improves with alcohol and propranolol and is made worse by anxiety.

29 A. This patient is most likely to be taking Levodopa for his Parkinson's. A side effect of this medication is chorea.

30 C. The term used to describe a sudden involuntary jerking of a single muscle group.

31 D. The term used to describe such a presentation. Botulinum helps to inhibit the release of acetylcholine from nerve endings into muscle.

32 E. The diagnosis is Parkinson's disease. Levodopa is the initial treatment of choice when symptoms are particularly disabling as in this case.

33 A. This patient has Parkinson's disease. The pathogenesis of this condition is primarily the result of depletion of dopamine containing neurones in the substantia nigra and basal ganglia.

34 C. Typical features of parkinsonism plus in which there is parkinsonism with additional features. This case is progressive supranuclear palsy.

35 A. Additional features include urinary incontinence.

36 B. Also commonly know as a petit mal seizure.

37 C. The presentation is that of a Jacksonian motor seizure. This is essentially a partial seizure which can lead to paralysis of involved limbs for several hours.

38 D. The diagnosis is a temporal lobe seizure due to experience of olfactory hallucinations. Visual hallucinations and experience of déjà vu are also common.

39 D. Sodium valproate is known to induce significant liver damage and hair loss.

40 A. A side effect of phenytoin is osteomalacia and folate deficiency.

41 C. Ethosuximide is known to cause 'night terrors' and rashes.

42 E. Diazepam given rectally is a useful alternative if intravenous access is difficult.

43 D. Blood glucose measurement should be taken immediately to ensure the patient is not hypoglycaemic. A CT scan should then be arranged to ensure there is no evidence of an intracranial haemorrhage.

44 A. The most likely diagnosis is a subarachnoid haemorrhage with raised intracranial pressure. A CT head scan is the initial investigation.

45 B. A yellow coloured supernatant is diagnostic of a subarachnoid haemorrhage and is due to lysis of red blood cells.

46 C. Subdural haematomas are often seen in elderly or alcoholic patients. Their atrophic brains make vessel rupture more likely.

47 E. The diagnosis is most likely to be an extradural haemorrhage due to temporal bone fracture and subsequent rupture of the middle meningeal artery.

48 D. Such neurological symptoms which improve within 24 hours are indicative of transient ischaemic attacks.

49 E. Transient global amnesia is associated with the vertebrobasilar vasculature and not the carotids.

50 B. The most likely diagnosis is a cerebral hemisphere infarct caused by occlusion of the middle cerebral artery.

51 D. The diagnosis is lateral medullary syndrome caused by occlusion of the posterior inferior cerebellar artery. Additional features may include palatal paralysis, nystagmus and Horner's syndrome.

52 A. The most likely diagnosis is an ischaemic stroke. A head CT scan is the initial investigation to exclude a haemorrhage, although an infarct may not be shown in the early stages. In the case of an infarct, carotid dopplers would then be performed as the bruit is indicative of stenosis and there is a potential for carotid endarterectomy.

53 E. Aspirin is the first line management following a cerebral infarct. He has presented too late to be considered for thrombolysis.

54 D. Opening eyes spontaneously = 4, Confused speech = 4, Withdrawing to pain = 4.

55 A. A scotoma is an area of depressed vision within the visual field. Such a finding is seen in lesions of the optic nerve which are commonly associated with demyelination as is the case with multiple sclerosis.

56 D. This is commonly seen in lesions of the temporal lobe.

57 A. Third nerve palsy results in pupillary dilatation.

58 D. The diagnosis is a third nerve palsy most likely due to a berry aneurysm arising in the posterior communicating artery.

59 C. Typical features of Ramsay Hunt syndrome. The condition results in a lower motor neurone facial palsy with herpetic vesicles in the external auditory meatus and soft palate.

60 B. This patient is experiencing vertigo as a result of gentamicin toxicity to the vestibular apparatus. Vertigo indicates a disturbance of the inner ear, eight cranial nerve or brainstem.

61 E. In pseudobulbar palsy the tongue is small and spastic. There are no notable fasciculations.

62 B. As multiple sclerosis may affect the cerebellum, horizontal nystagmus is typically seen.

Extended matching questions

Theme: Cranial nerve lesions

1 C. Characteristic features of a third nerve palsy.

2 G. Additional features include undue sensitivity to sound.

3 D. Typical presentation of damage to the trochlear nerve.

4 B. This visual loss is commonly known as a scotoma which may occur centrally or paracentrally.

5 E. Such lesions may also be associated with jaw deviation to the side of the lesion.

Theme: Diseases of the peripheral nerves

1 F. Also seen in patients with hypothyroidism. Carpal tunnel syndrome may also be associated with sensory loss of the palm and radial three and a half fingers.

2 D. Typical presentation of Charcot–Marie–Tooth disease.

3 E. Additional features include bowel and bladder weakness.

4 B. Such deficiency may lead to Wernicke–Korsakoff syndrome.

5 A. Isoniazid is associated with vitamin B6 deficiency.

Theme: Diseases of the muscle

1 J. Duchenne muscular dystrophy is an X-linked recessive condition caused by a mutation on chromosome 21. Death is common in the late teens.

2 C. Additional features include fatigability of extra ocular muscles and muscles of facial expression.

3 D. Additional features include cardiomyopathy, glucose intolerance and hypogonadism.

4 E. The myotonia is often made worse during rest.

5 A. An autosomal recessive condition which can progress to severe disability within 20 years time.

Theme: Epilepsy

1 A. Tongue biting is often seen in such cases.

2 B. Typical presentation of petit mal seizures.

3 D. This is a simple partial seizure which can lead to paralysis of the involved limbs for several hours.

4 A. Carbamazepine or sodium valproate are also useful agents.

5 E. Additional features include olfactory and visual hallucinations.

Theme: Extrapyramidal diseases

1 D. Typical presentation of Parkinsonism plus. There is often a poor response to levodopa in these cases.

2 H. This is usually caused by infarction or haemorrhage in the contralateral subthalamic nucleus.

3 G. Typical features include chorea, personality change and dementia.

4 J. Classic description of a tic.

5 B. Sites typically affected include the optic nerves, the brainstem, the cerebellum and the cervical spinal cord.

Answers **Haematology**

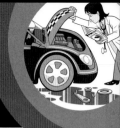

Single best answer

1 D. The diagnosis is polycythaemia vera based on the blood count, splenomegaly and raised red cell volume. This is usually managed via venesection in the first instance. There is no absolute cure.

2 C. 'Tear drop'-shaped red cells are found in myelofibrosis and can also be found in other myeloproliferative disorders, pernicious anaemia, thalassaemia, myeloid metaplasia, and some haemolytic anaemias.

3 A. This patient is experiencing an anaphylactic reaction best managed with 0.5 mg adrenaline intramuscularly.

4 D. Factor VII initiates the clotting process following tissue damage.

5 A. This patient is likely to be suffering from autoimmune thrombocytopenic purpura. Platelet count is the first line investigation.

6 D. This patient is suffering from haemophilia A which is due to deficiency of factor VIII. The history suggests mild haemophilia and the treatment in this case is replacement of factor VIII for bleeding episodes.

7 E. Vitamin K is necessary for the activity of prothrombin (II), VII, IX and X. Absorption of vitamin K and other fat soluble vitamins will be impaired by cholestasis and hence lead to impaired coagulation by altering activity of these factors.

8 A. The diagnosis is a probable deep vein thrombosis. Doppler ultrasound is useful for ileofemoral thrombosis. Calf vein thrombosis is best assessed by venography.

9 C. Activated partial thromboplastin time is used for monitoring of unfractionated heparin. Prothrombin time and INR is utilised for warfarin monitoring.

10 D. The warfarin should be stopped and reinstituted when the INR has fallen within the therapeutic range. Other measures are usually only necessary if the INR is very high (>9) or if there is bleeding.

11 C. Auer rods are characteristic of acute myeloid leukaemia.

12 E. Hyponatraemia does not occur in acute tumour lysis syndrome.

13 D. All trans retinoic acid is proven to induce remission in this form of leukaemia.

14 A. The Philadelphia chromosome is invariably present in chronic myeloid leukaemia but can occasionally occur in acute lymphoblastic leukaemia.

15 C. In addition to the central nervous system this form of leukaemia may affect the testes in males.

16 C. Tyrosine kinase inhibitors such as Imatinib are the initial treatment of choice for chronic myeloid leukaemia and has better outcomes than alpha interferon plus cytarabine which was the previous standard of care.

17 D. Smear cells are characteristic of chronic lymphocytic leukaemia. They reflect fragility and distortion of B-CLL cells while the film is being made.

18 E. This patient is likely to be suffering from Hodgkin's disease which is most appropriately diagnosed by lymph node biopsy and histology.

19 D. Characteristic presentation of Hodgkin's disease.

20 B. Sternberg Reed cells are malignant B lymphocytes and are diagnostic of Hodgkin's disease.

21 E. Additional 'B' symptoms include fever and weight loss.

22 C. Age is not an important factor when determining treatment in the vast majority of cases.

23 E. The gastrointestinal tract may be affected but not in all cases.

24 D. MALT lymphoma typically affects the stomach.

25 C. Burkitt's lymphoma typically affects African children and can result in jaw tumours.

26 B. Key features of multiple myeloma. Additional features include gangrene and bleeding.

27 D. The initial test is protein electrophoresis which will reveal the presence of a monoclonal protein ('M' bands). A bone marrow examination showing 10% or more clonal bone marrow plasma cells will be necessary to make the diagnosis.

28 C. Heavy menstruation is known to cause iron deficiency anaemia.

29 B. This patient has iron deficiency anaemia in view of her low ferritin. The blood film will show all except macrocytosis.

30 A. This is commonly seen in chronic illnesses, such as Crohn's disease, renal failure and tuberculosis. Laboratory findings include a low serum iron, low serum iron binding capacity and an increased or normal serum ferritin. Treatment is of the underlying cause.

31 C. Vitamin B12 deficiency is commonly seen in vegans who do not consume animal products.

32 E. In view of her autoimmune thyroid disease, age and macrocytosis the most likely diagnosis is pernicious anaemia, an autoimmune disease. She will be vitamin B12 deficient but the key to the diagnosis is the presence of intrinsic factor antibodies which are more specific for the disease than parietal cell auto antibodies.

33 C. All of these could cause vitamin B12 deficiency but the history makes coeliac disease the most likely.

34 C. Megaloblastic anaemia is seen in vitamin B12 and folate deficiency. In this case the cause is not clear so replacement with both vitamin B12 and folate is given pending the results for measurement of vitamin B12 and serum folate. Folate alone has been shown to worsen the neurological complications of vitamin B12 deficiency.

35 C. The reticulocyte count is increased in haemolytic anaemia.

36 D. The clinical features are characteristic of Beta Thalassaemia major.

37 B. This patient is experiencing a sickle-cell crisis. As her oxygen saturation is currently within normal range, analgesia would be the most suitable management step.

38 A. Systemic lupus erythematosus is associated with autoimmune haemolytic anaemia. Coomb's test is diagnostic in this form of anaemia.

39 D. The diagnosis is cold antibody haemolysis which is best managed by avoidance of cold exposure.

40 A. Warm antibody haemolytic anaemia is characterised by IgG antibodies. Cold antibody haemolytic anaemia is characterised by IgM antibodies.

Extended matching questions

Theme: Anaemia

1 C. Such a form of anaemia is best treated supportively with red cell and platelet transfusion in addition to antibiotic use for infections associated with neutropenia.

2 I. Common in Northern Europe, this form of anaemia can result in splenomegaly and leg ulcers. Treatment is usually a splenectomy.

3 J. Cigar-shaped red blood cells are characteristic of hereditary elliptocytosis. Treatment is usually not required.

4 F. Haemolysis is the result of oxidant red cell damage. In addition to fava beans drugs such as sulphonamides may precipitate haemolysis.

5 D. This condition may eventually progress to myelodysplasia and leukaemia.

Theme: Lymphadenopathy

1 A. Epstein–Barr virus is typically transmitted in saliva. In rare cases there may be splenic rupture, myocarditis and meningitis.

2 F. The virus may be transmitted sexually or via contaminated blood products in the main. HIV is an RNA virus which binds to CD4 cells via gp120 to cause cellular damage.

3 C. Characteristic description of a lymphoma.

4 D. Genetic factors such as the Philadelphia chromosome are responsible for the majority of chronic myeloid leukaemia cases. Environmental factors include radiation exposure and drugs such as chemotherapy.

5 B. Additional features may include retinitis, loss of visual acuity and orbital pain.

Theme: **Splenomegaly**

1 A. This is characteristic of schistosomiasis, which is most prevalent in Africa.

2 H. Characteristic features of Kala azar. Additional features include pyrexia, sweats, a burning sensation in the feet and joint pain.

3 D. Four main malarial parasites exist. These include *Plasmodium falciparum*, *vivax*, *ovale* and *malariae*. Clinical features of falciparum malaria include impaired consciousness, uraemia, respiratory distress syndrome and splenic rupture.

4 G. A classic description of Gaucher's disease of which there exists three types. Type 2 and type 3 have a propensity to involve the central nervous system.

5 J. Additional features may include epistaxis and bruising. Ciprofloxacin is the mainstay form of treatment.

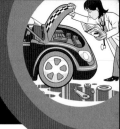
Single best answer

1 A. Sick sinus syndrome is characterised by a time interval of greater than 2 seconds between consecutive P waves. The very slow P rate and relatively stable ventricular rate suggests a sinoatrial problem rather than an AV nodal problem. Thromboembolism is a feature and patients often require anticoagulation.

2 C. Also known as Wenckebach's phenomenon. This arrhythmia is characterised by an increasing PR interval until the P wave no longer conducts to the ventricles.

3 B. First degree heart block is the result of delayed atrioventricular conduction and is characterised by a PR interval greater than 0.22 seconds.

4 D. Second degree block is characterised by an intermittent failure or interruption of AV conduction but there is no increasing PR interval as is the case with Mobitz Type 1 block.

5 E. Typical symptoms include blackouts and dizzy spells. Pacemaker insertion is the mainstay form of treatment.

6 A. This is atrial flutter with 2:1 block and characterised by sawtooth flutter waves on the ECG.

7 E. The diagnosis is atrial flutter of recent onset and treated with electrical cardioversion in the first instance.

8 A. The diagnosis is atrial fibrillation. Current NICE (National Institute of Health and Clinical Excellence) guidelines state beta blockers are the initial choice of management for rate control.

9 C. The diagnosis is a supraventricular tachycardia (SVT). Carotid sinus massage is helpful in the acute situation. Other manoeuvres may include the Valsalva manoeuvre. Adenosine is used in the treatment of SVT but is contraindicated in this patient because of asthma.

10 A. The diagnosis is pulseless electrical activity due to hypovolaemia. This is a non shockable rhythm. Administration of colloid, saline or blood would be the next most appropriate step in management followed by adrenaline 1 mg IV.

11 A. Typical features of mitral stenosis. Additional signs include a malar flush and tapping apex beat.

12 B. Typical features of mitral regurgitation. Additional signs include a displaced apex beat.

13 C. Additional signs would include a slow rising carotid pulse.

14 D. Additional signs would include a collapsing pulse, a displaced apex beat and a mid diastolic murmur over the cardiac apex.

15 C. Typical features of tricuspid regurgitation. Abdominal examination is likely to reveal an enlarged pulsatile liver.

16 B. An echo is the first line investigation in the diagnosis of cardiac murmurs.

17 E. The diagnosis is mitral stenosis. A widened carina on the chest X-ray is normally seen.

18 B. The echocardiogram is the most useful investigation and may show regional wall abnormalities with ischaemia, valve abnormalities and pericardial thickening. A chest X-ray will usually, but not always, show typical features of heart failure but will not usually demonstrate the cause.

19 C. The patient is suffering from left sided heart failure. Chest X-ray features include fluid in the right horizontal fissure seen as a white line running over the anterior end of the 4th rib. There is no horizontal fissure in the left lung as there are only two lobes.

20 A. Ischaemic heart disease is the most common cause of heart failure in the western world.

21 E. The diagnosis is heart failure. Current guidelines state ACE inhibitors are typically the first line treatment in heart failure. However as this patient is severely fluid overloaded, diuretics such as furosemide would be the first line of treatment.

22 B. This class of drug is known to cause hyperkalemia.

23 D. The diagnosis is pulmonary oedema. Furosemide is the most appropriate treatment.

GTN (glyceryl trinitrate) may be used if he does not respond to diuretics to reduce the cardiac preload.

24 E. Low intake of folic acid is a risk factor for ischaemic heart disease.

25 C. Such a syndrome is thought to be due in part to an abnormal coronary microcirculation. Angiograms are always normal.

26 B. The patient is experiencing angina which is best treated by GTN in the first instance.

27 E. Enoxaparin 1 mg/kg twice daily is the recommended dose in patients with evidence of acute coronary syndrome

28 E. Typical ECG changes of a posterior infarct.

29 A. Troponin is the most appropriate investigation in individuals with chest pain as it is highly specific and sensitive for cardiac damage.

30 D. Aspirin 300 mg is the recommended immediate management in a suspected myocardial infarction.

31 D. Pericarditis is an early complication of a myocardial infarction and typically occurs within the first 2–4 days.

32 D. This is the most likely organism to cause infective endocarditis in intravenous drug abusers and those with central venous lines.

33 A. This is the most likely offending organism associated with dental diseases or procedures.

34 A. A splenic abscess is more likely to be due to embolisation of vegetations of fibrin and platelets.

35 E. The most likely diagnosis is infective endocarditis typically confirmed by three sets of blood cultures in the first instance.

36 A. Classic features of a dilated cardiomyopathy.

37 B. Additional features include a jerky carotid pulse and an ejection systolic murmur.

38 A. Classic presentation of pericarditis. Management is usually with NSAIDs or corticosteroids.

39 B. This patient has developed a pericardial effusion. Echo is diagnostic.

40 C. According to current guidelines ACE inhibitors are the first line management of hypertension in diabetic patients.

41 C. Additional features include 'cotton wool' exudates.

Extended matching questions

Theme: Chest pain

1 A. Typical presentation of angina pectoris.

2 C. Classic features of a myocardial infarction. Additional features would include sweating, breathlessness, nausea and vomiting.

3 D. There may also be unequal blood pressure in both arms.

4 H. Classic description of costochondritis.

5 B. Pain may also radiate to the neck and shoulders.

Theme: Drugs

1 E. Captopril is an ACE inhibitor which can lead to a cough due to inhibition of bradykinin metabolism. Other side effects include renal failure and angioedema.

2 E. ACE inhibitors such as captopril can affect renal function in patients with renovascular disease. This is due to elimination of efferent vasoconstriction which leads to a decrease in the glomerular filtration rate.

3 D. Typical side effects of calcium channel blockers.

4 C. Aspirin is regarded as the gold standard in the management of acute coronary syndrome.

5 A. This is due to bronchoconstrictive and vasoconstrictive effects.

Theme: Clinical features of cardiac disease

1 D. Classic features of mitral regurgitation.

2 E. Additional features would include Roth's spots and Osler's nodes.

3 F. The pink coloured rings are characteristic of erythema marginatum seen typically in rheumatic fever. One would also expect to suffer from arthritis and cardiac murmurs.

4 A. Classic presentation of aortic stenosis.

5 I. Additional features include chest pain and dyspnoea.

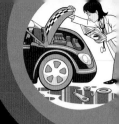

Single best answer

1 B.   *Helicobacter pylori* causes a decrease in somatostatin levels. Additional effects include an increase in pepsinogen 1 and urease.

2 C.   The diagnosis is gastro-oesophageal reflux disease which is usually investigated by upper gastrointestinal endoscopy as a first line. However, in patients less than 55 years and without alarm symptoms or signs it is reasonable to have a trial of treatment before proceeding with investigations.

3 D.   Proton pump inhibitors such as lansoprazole or omeprazole are usually first choice.

4 A.   A classic description of achalasia. This is a motility disorder associated with aperistalsis and failure of relaxation of the lower oesophageal sphincter. The tapered portion of the oesophagus is commonly referred to as a beak deformity.

5 C.   A 'corkscrew' appearance is diagnostic of diffuse oesophageal spasm. Treatment often involves the use of calcium channel blockers.

6 E.   Gastro-oesophageal reflux disease is a risk factor for adenocarcinoma and not squamous cell carcinoma.

7 C.   Management of *Helicobacter pylori* infection involves a proton pump inhibitor and two antibiotics. Common regimens include omeprazole, metronidazole and clarithromycin, or omeperazole, amoxicillin and clarithromycin.

8 D.   The diagnosis is most likely gastric cancer. The peri-orbital skin rash is classic of dermatomyositis which is associated with an underlying malignancy in some cases. An upper gastrointestinal endoscopy is the most appropriate investigation.

9 E.   Tar-coloured stool is commonly known as melaena and signifies an upper gastrointestinal bleed. The most common cause of such a bleed is a peptic ulcer.

10 A.   Severe vomiting often leads to a tear in the oesophagus and a subsequent bleed.

11 C.   Diclofenac is a non steroidal anti-inflammatory drug and can cause peptic ulceration which may be complicated by bleeding or perforation.

12 D.   This patient is haemodynamically unstable and hence the first line treatment would be intravenous access and urgent fluid resuscitation with saline or O negative blood.

13 A.   The first line investigation for a PR bleed is always a rectal examination but it is likely he will need to go on and have one or more of the listed investigations.

14 C.   This patient has iron deficiency anaemia and the initial investigation is an upper and lower gastrointestinal endoscopy ('top and tail') to look for a source of GI blood loss such as a malignancy.

15 E.   Coeliac disease is the most likely as it is common (1% of the population) and causes these symptoms. Other listed diagnoses are far less common, other than IBS which does not cause iron and folate deficiency.

16 D.   There is often absent or stunted small intestinal villi in coeliac disease with elongation of crypts.

17 A.   The first line investigation to prove coeliac disease is endoscopy and biopsy.

18 C.   These symptoms suggest small bowel bacterial overgrowth following recent surgery. The hydrogen breath test helps to demonstrate the presence of such organisms. Upon ingestion of glucose the bacteria will metabolise the sugar and produce hydrogen which can then be subsequently measured in exhaled air.

19 A.   Smoking increases the risk of developing Crohn's disease.

20 D.   Skip lesions are characteristic of Crohn's disease.

21 E.   Tachypnoea is not a characteristic of an acute attack of ulcerative colitis. Additional features would include anaemia and a low serum albumin.

135

22 A. Gall bladder calculi are not related to disease activity.

23 E. Serum sodium is not a marker of an acute exacerbation of Crohn's disease.

24 B. In cases of acute severe colitis intravenous hydrocortisone is the first line treatment with ciclosporin being considered if patients do not respond.

25 A. His symptoms suggest a flare and steroids are the most appropriate treatment.

26 A. Colon cancer is more common in ulcerative colitis.

27 C. The most likely diagnosis is acute diverticulitis. Abdominal and pelvic CT scan is the most appropriate investigation.

28 B. A high serum potassium is not a cause of constipation. Potassium is in fact known to aid bowel motility.

29 B. As the tumour has extended through the bowel wall and not involved lymph nodes the diagnosis is Dukes' stage B.

30 C. The staging investigations suggest Dukes' stage C cancer. Surgery in addition to post operative chemotherapy is the most effective form of management.

31 D. Although dietary and lifestyle factors are thought to play an aetiological role, family history is the most important aetiological factor in this case.

32 A. An ileoscopy would assess for recurrent Crohn's disease which is the most likely diagnosis.

33 D. Sepsis is common with TPN. To confirm a source, both peripheral and line cultures should be taken and TPN stopped until cultures are deemed negative.

34 A. This patient has developed jaundice. Following liver biochemistry an ultrasound scan is the initial investigation to assess for biliary duct dilatation.

35 B. Hepatitis A is commonly due to ingestion of contaminated water or food such as shellfish. Symptoms such as abdominal pain, diarrhoea and dark urine are characteristic of the condition.

36 C. Elevated aminotransferases are diagnostic of hepatocyte damage. Hepatitis B is commonly due to intravenous drug abuse and can lead to joint stiffness and skin rashes in certain cases.

37 E. This patient has developed jaundice as a result of hepatitis C. Hepatitis C is known to cause glomerulonephritis which explains this patient's haematuria.

38 D. This patient most probably has a diagnosis of hepatitis A which is commonly due to consumption of contaminated food such as shellfish or clams.

39 C. Grade 3 encephalopathy comprises features of drowsiness, stupor and no evidence of communication.

40 B. The suspected diagnosis is autoimmune hepatitis which is more common in patients with other autoimmune conditions. This condition is associated with high titres of antinuclear antibodies.

41 D. The best assessment of liver function in cirrhotic patients is prothrombin time.

42 E. The prognosis of cirrhosis is based on 5 variables known as Child's grading. These include encephalopathy, ascites, prothrombin time, serum albumin and serum bilirubin.

43 A. With any gastrointestinal bleed an urgent endoscopy is the most appropriate initial management following adequate resuscitation of the patient.

44 B. Meig's syndrome is an example of a transudate.

45 C. This patient has developed ascites. The initial management is with diuretics such as spironolactone and sodium restriction.

46 B. This patient has developed spontaneous bacterial peritonitis which is a complication of ascites in chronic liver disease. The most common organism in this condition is *Escherichia coli*.

47 E. The diagnosis is hepatic encephalopathy, confirmed by features of asterixis, fetor hepaticus and confusion. The diagnosis is usually clinical but an EEG will show characteristic changes if there is diagnostic uncertainty.

48 D. The history suggests primary biliary cirrhosis, a condition known to affect middle aged women. Serum AMAs are the first line investigation.

49 E. The diagnosis in this case is haemochromatosis based on the history and examination. From the listed options serum ferritin is the most appropriate diagnostic tool.

50 C. The diagnosis is alcoholic hepatitis in view of the presence of mallory bodies. Stopping alcohol completely is the mainstay form of treatment in order to prevent the development of alcoholic cirrhosis.

51 D. This patient is likely to be suffering from a primary hepatocellular carcinoma in view of his weight loss, presence of ascites and raised alpha fetoprotein level. Ultrasound scan or CT is the most appropriate diagnostic tool.

52 E. The clinical diagnosis is acute cholecystitis most appropriately investigated by abdominal ultrasound scan.

53 A. This patient has developed acute pancreatitis. Hyperglycaemia is a well recognised complication of this condition.

54 D. The diagnosis is chronic pancreatitis. As a result of pancreatic lipase secretion reduction, this patient has developed steatorrhoea. Chronic pancreatitis is most appropriately investigated by abdominal CT scan.

55 B. Pancreatic carcinoma has a poor prognosis. This lady is elderly and frail with metastatic disease and therefore is likely to have palliative treatment only.

Extended matching questions

Theme: Hepatobiliary disorders

1 G. This condition is associated with a triad of skin pigmentation, diabetes and hepatomegaly. Treatment is with venesection initially weekly and then less frequently to maintain iron depletion.

2 B. This disorder can result in liver cirrhosis and emphysema. There is no specific treatment available.

3 J. Such a disorder is most appropriately diagnosed by the presence of anti mitochondrial antibodies. Treatment plans include the use of ursodeoxycholic acid and cholestyramine to help relieve pruritus.

4 A. Wilson's disease is associated with an error of copper metabolism. Treatment consists of chelating agents such as penicillamine or trientene.

5 F. Primary sclerosing cholangitis is diagnosed following a liver biopsy which demonstrates evidence of polymorph infiltration of bile ducts. An ERCP may also be useful in such cases and may demonstrate a bead like appearance within the bile ducts as a result of stricture formation.

Theme: Gastrointestinal bleeding

1 C. Additional symptoms may include peri anal irritation and itch. Treatment involves the use of sclerosant injections, elastic band ligation or surgical resection.

2 A. This is a classic presentation of a Mallory Weiss tear. Forceful vomiting has led to a tear in the oesophagus and a subsequent bleed.

3 B. The aetiology of this condition is unknown but there is a strong association with underlying cardiac disease particularly aortic stenosis. Treatment typically involves the use of diathermy or surgical resection.

4 G. Classic description of reflux disease.

5 E. The gram negative bacterium is most probably *Helicobacter pylori* which is commonly associated with both gastric and duodenal ulcers.

Theme: Drugs

1 D. Acamprosate is known to help reduce one's craving experienced by alcohol dependent patients. It is thought to interact with glutamate and GABA neurotransmitters to restore neuronal excitation and inhibition balance.

2 F. Acute severe exacerbations involve the use of intravenous steroids in almost all cases.

3 B. In view of his stroke this patient is likely to have been prescribed aspirin. Aspirin is an anti platelet drug and can increase the risk of gastrointestinal bleeding.

4 A. This patient is likely to be suffering from gastro-oesophageal reflux disease. Agents such as proton pump inhibitors or alginate containing antacids are beneficial in such cases.

5 E. The diagnosis is Crohn's disease in view of histological findings. Mesalazine induces remission in this condition.

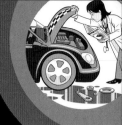

Single best answer

1 C. The correct term used to describe this area.

2 D. The term used to describe this finding.

3 A. The diagnosis is acute appendicitis. Abdominal CT scan or ultrasound are the most preferred investigative tools. Abdominal X-ray is of no diagnostic benefit.

4 A. The 'drip and suck' technique. Patients are severely dehydrated and require intravenous saline for adequate fluid resuscitation.

5 A. This patient is likely to have acute pancreatitis best diagnosed by an abdominal CT scan.

6 E. An arterial PO_2 of less than 10 kPa is an indicator of severity.

7 B. The term most appropriately used to describe this finding.

8 A. Ascites is not a complication of acute pancreatitis.

9 E. The diagnosis is renal colic best assessed by an intravenous urogram.

10 B. This patient is demonstrating evidence of gall bladder disease best diagnosed by abdominal ultrasound in the first instance.

11 E. Presentation of a ruptured abdominal aortic aneurysm. Surgery is the most appropriate intervention.

12 C. Presentation of lower limb ischaemia on the background of atrial fibrillation. In view of her satisfactory blood pressure and oxygen saturation an emergency embolectomy would be the next most appropriate management step.

13 A. The diagnosis is acute diverticulitis. Additional features would include rectal bleeding and altered bowel habit. Such a condition is best diagnosed by abdominal CT scan.

14 D. The diagnosis is cholecystitis in view of his right upper quadrant pain, pyrexia and elevated inflammatory markers. The mainstay form of treatment is regular analgesia and antibiotic use.

15 C. Additional features may include menstrual cycle irregularities and micturition abnormalities.

16 E. Additional features would include swelling of the testicle and no relief of pain upon elevation of the scrotum. This is unlike epididymitis where elevation may help improve the pain.

17 A. Classical presentation of epididymitis. Antibiotics and analgesia are the mainstay form of treatment.

Extended matching questions

Theme: Acute abdomen

1 H. A classic presentation of bowel obstruction.

2 J. Free gas on an erect chest X-ray is diagnostic of a perforation.

3 C. Typical presentation of renal colic.

4 B. An abnormal amylase together with abdominal tenderness are key features of pancreatitis.

5 F. The diagnosis is a dissecting aortic aneurysm in view of symptomatology and a widened mediastinum.

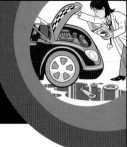
Single best answer

1 A. A classic presentation of an indirect inguinal hernia. Such hernias pass through the internal ring lateral to the inferior epigastric artery, along the canal to emerge at the external ring above the pubic crest and tubercle.

2 B. A description of a direct inguinal hernia. Such hernias bulge through the posterior wall of the canal, medial to the inferior epigastric artery. They do not protrude into the scrotum.

3 D. Indirect inguinal hernias are typically lateral to the inferior epigastric vessels.

4 C. Femoral hernias are 4 times more common in women and present below and lateral to the pubic tubercle.

5 A. A classic description of an umbilical hernia. Such hernias are at great risk of strangulation.

6 A. Epigastric hernias typically present in the midline and are often tender and irreducible.

7 D. Risk factors for incisional hernia formation include age, diabetes, obesity, malnutrition, jaundice and sepsis to name but a few.

8 C. Spigelian hernias present as lumps at the lateral margin of the rectus sheath. Strangulation or obstruction often occur.

9 B. Obturator hernias are typically seen in elderly women. The hernia occurs through the obturator canal within the pelvis so the patient often presents with small bowel obstruction. There may also be pain along the medial aspect of the thigh due to pressure on the obturator nerve.

Extended matching questions

Theme: **Hernia**

1 G. A partially obstructed hernia which can lead to bowel perforation through ischaemia.

2 J. Such hernias occur when part of the stomach or intestine protrude into the chest cavity through a defect in the diaphragm.

3 I. Such hernias are often difficult to distinguish from inguinal hernias and may lead to strangulation or obstruction.

4 B. Such hernias are essentially a combination of an indirect and direct hernia.

5 A. A classic description of a direct inguinal hernia.

Answers Vascular surgery

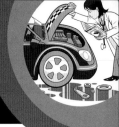

Single best answer

1 A. Back pain is characteristic of a thoracic aortic aneurysm. Swallowing impairment is typical due to compression of the cervical oesophagus. This is, however, rare.

2 E. This artery is commonly damaged in abdominal aortic aneurysm repair and is most likely responsible for paraplegia post operatively.

3 C. The abdominal aorta is considered aneurysmal if its diameter exceeds three centimetres.

4 B. The first most appropriate investigation is ultrasound. CT scanning is only useful later to determine whether endovascular or open repair is appropriate.

5 D. Over resuscitation with fluids only serves to increase bleeding into the abdomen. A systolic pressure of 80 mmHg is more than sufficient.

6 C. Rupture is rare and occurs in less than 5% of cases.

7 D. Typical presentation of a mycotic aneurysm. Such aneurysms arise from infection within the vessel wall.

8 E. Such aneurysms occur when an artery has been damaged. In this case the femoral artery has been punctured for an angiogram but has failed to seal.

9 A. Lower back pain is not a typical feature of lower limb ischaemia.

10 B. The diagnosis is intermittent claudication which is most likely investigated via measurement of ankle brachial pressure index. This is often reduced by approximately 60–70%.

11 D. Risk factor modification is always the first line management of intermittent claudication, in this case, hypertension. Drug therapy and surgery is rarely common practice in the first instance.

12 C. Pulses are usually present in individuals with neuropathic ulcers.

13 E. The hypoglossal nerve may be damaged as it crosses the internal carotid artery.

14 A. Hand-held Doppler helps to confirm saphenofemoral and saphenopopliteal incompetence. Other useful tests include venography and plethysmography but these are rarely needed.

15 D. Compression stockings are the initial choice of management. Surgery is a useful second option. Laser therapy and radio frequency ablation are considered if the above options have failed.

16 B. The diagnosis here is most likely to be lymphoedema with treatment being in the form of compression stockings in the main.

17 C. Arterial leg ulcers feel more comfortable hanging down.

Extended matching questions

Theme: **Vascular disorders**

1 E. Also known as Buerger's disease. This condition is characterized by segmental thrombotic occlusions of small and medium sized vessels in both upper and lower limbs.

2 F. Treatment typically involves avoidance of cold and stopping smoking. Medical treatment includes the use of nifedipine.

3 I. This is essentially recurrent episodes of superficial thrombophlebitis which may also precede clinical manifestations of malignancy.

4 A. Typical features of an abdominal aortic aneurysm. Surgery is typically indicated for aneurysms which are symptomatic or those which are asymptomatic but greater than 5 cm.

5 C. Diagnosis is often confirmed via chest X-ray which typically shows a widened mediastinum. Management involves surgery and urgent blood pressure control.

145

Answers Breast disease

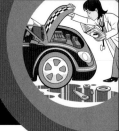

Single best answer

1 A. A classic description of localised fibroadenosis. Triple assessment would be required to establish the diagnosis.

2 D. This lady has a fibroadenoma, commonly nick-named 'breast mice', due to their mobility within the breast tissue.

3 E. Breast cysts are discrete mobile lumps which produce a straw coloured fluid on aspiration.

4 A. Mammary duct ectasia presents with nipple retraction as a result of fibrosis and a milky or dirty green discharge. However, formal triple assessment must be undertaken to exclude malignancy.

5 B. A description of a duct papilloma. The discharge may be serous or blood stained.

6 C. Breast cancer is rare under the age of 35. Individuals greater than 50 years of age are at a greater risk.

7 D. BRCA1 on chromosome 17Q and BRCA2 on chromosome 13Q are associated with breast cancer.

8 A. In the UK women between the ages of 50 and 64 are called every 3 years for screening.

9 C. Stage 3 comprises of any sized tumour, involvement of fixed ipsilateral axillary nodes or ipsilateral supraclavicular or infraclavicular nodes and no evidence of distant metastasis. It may also comprise of any sized tumour, no palpable or palpable lymph nodes and no evidence of distant metastasis.

10 B. This is a stage 2 cancer with a 5-year survival rate of 71%.

11 A. Ductal cancers are the most common breast cancers with a frequency of 80%.

12 D. Ultrasound helps to distinguish a solid mass from a cystic mass and is preferable to mammography in women under the age of 35 years in whom the breast tissue is very dense.

13 A. This is a locally advanced breast cancer (stage 3) and is best treated with neoadjuvant chemotherapy, followed, if possible, by breast conserving surgery and axillary clearance. As it is oestrogen receptor negative tamoxifen would be of no use. Herceptin would only be utilised if the cancer were HER2-positive.

14 E. Paget's disease commonly presents as an eczematous eruption of the nipple.

15 C. A classic description of a Phylloides tumour. Histologically the tumour would have a characteristic leaf like appearance.

Extended matching questions

Theme: **Management of breast cancer**

1 B. Also known as herceptin, this drug interferes with the attachment of human epidermal growth factor to Her 2 and thus prevents the division and growth of breast cancer cells.

2 C. Additional side effects include flushes, hot sweats and irregular periods.

3 D. Such drugs prevent the conversion of androgens into oestrogen which is needed for the growth of breast cancer.

4 B. Other common side effects include diarrhoea, tumour pain and headaches.

5 A. This agent is also commonly associated with tumours of the kidney.

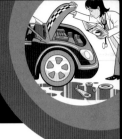

Single best answer

1 D. Likely diagnosis of acute osteomyelitis most commonly due to *Staphylococcus aureus* in over 80% of cases.

2 A. MRI has become the gold standard investigation replacing fluid aspiration for culture. Plain limb X-rays may be normal for up to 10 days.

3 E. A tumour derived from osteoblasts. The 'sun ray' like appearance is due to the formation of bony spicules.

4 B. Classic presentation of acromioclavicular osteoarthritis. Excision of the outer end of the clavicle may help to relieve symptoms.

5 A. This is a common problem to affect the shoulder best treated with NSAIDs or steroid injections.

6 C. Typical presentation of a rotator cuff tear. Usually associated with traumatic injury or dislocation. Management is usually through surgery in the young.

7 C. The diagnosis is tennis elbow or lateral epicondylitis best treated with NSAIDs initially.

8 B. Usual features of ulnar nerve neuropathy.

9 A. Classic presentation of a radial nerve injury.

10 B. This condition is typically due to thickening and shortening of the palmar fascia which becomes adherent to the skin. As a result the ring and little finger develop a fixed flexion deformity.

11 E. Results from localised thickening of the flexor tendon with associated sheath narrowing causing the finger to catch as it is flexed.

12 C. The diagnosis is most likely to be cauda equina syndrome. MRI is the gold standard investigation in such cases.

13 A. Plain X-ray is the best choice investigation from the listed options.

14 C. Anterior cruciate ligament rupture is the most likely cause in approximately 40% of cases.

15 C. Typical presentation of an anterior cruciate ligament injury. It is usually detected in approximately 70% of cases.

16 E. Here the tibia has been forced posteriorly resulting in such an injury.

17 B. Female sex is a risk factor for developmental dysplasia of the hip.

18 D. As the child is over 6 months this is the most suitable management. Before 6 months a splint is typically used.

19 D. This is a late complication of fractures.

20 D. Callus formation is usually visible within 3 weeks.

21 B. Typical presentation of Perthes' disease.

22 C. Usual findings of a slipped upper femoral epiphysis best treated with surgery.

Extended matching questions

Theme: **Fractures**

1 E. Classic history of a distal radius fracture. Associated with a backward angulation and displacement producing a dinner fork wrist.

2 C. Radial nerve injury may lead to a wrist drop. Immobilization is the mainstay form of treatment.

3 H. This occurs just below the femoral head.

4 D. Scaphoid fractures result in tenderness on direct pressure approximately 2 cm distal to Lister's tubercle of the radius and on proximal pressure on the extended thumb. If one suspects this fracture an additional oblique scaphoid view should be requested.

5 H. Presents with external rotation and adduction of the leg. Medial femoral circumflex artery involvement may lead to ischaemic necrosis of the femoral head.

Theme: **Fracture complications**

1 I. Hip fractures are commonly associated with the development of pneumonia. The severity of such a condition is based on the CURB 65 score which assesses the presence of confusion, serum urea, respiratory rate, blood pressure and age.

2 H. Classic features of a fat embolism.

3 D. Non union is commoner in cortical bone rather than in cancellous bone. Predisposing factors include malignancy and infection.

4 B. This complication is associated with fluid loss and acute tubular necrosis as a result of myoglobin release. An urgent fasciotomy may be required.

5 E. Classic description of malunion. The resulting deformity may be of length, angulation or rotation.

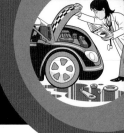

Single best answer

1 B. Presentation is usually during the second or third decade of life. Surgery is the mainstay form of management.

2 C. This cyst is typically smooth and mobile. Diagnosis is often by fine needle aspiration which produces a creamy coloured fluid.

3 D. Auscultation may often reveal a bruit. Surgical excision is the preferred treatment option.

4 C. A plain X-ray may help to reveal a stone in the parotid duct. Treatment is with mouth care, rehydration and antibiotics.

5 B. A benign tumour which may undergo malignant transformation.

6 E. This is a benign tumour which may occur bilaterally in approximately 10% of cases.

7 E. Two episodes of sore throat per year is not an indication for tonsillectomy according to the Scottish Intercollegiate Guidelines Network (SIGN).

8 A. Typical presentation of otitis externa. Management involves antibiotics topically in mild cases.

9 B. Rare after the age of 5. *Haemophilus influenzae* is the main organism responsible for such a condition in approximately 40% of cases. Complications include effusion or scarring of the tympanic membrane.

10 E. This is typically administered for a 7–10 day period.

11 D. This is essentially otitis media with effusion and typically occurs between the age of 2 and 6. In over 90% of cases the effusion resolves spontaneously.

12 C. This condition results in unilateral sensorineural hearing loss and tinnitus. Surgery is the mainstay form of treatment.

13 A. Antihistamines have been shown to decrease middle ear labyrinth excitability and block conduction in the middle ear vestibular cerebellar pathways which primarily aids in reducing vertigo.

14 D. In view of his haemodynamic instability and ongoing blood loss, intravenous access for urgent fluid resuscitation (in this case with blood), is the initial step in management.

15 E. Oral antihistamines may be added following steroid usage. Surgery is often the last resort.

16 A. This fracture is a low transverse fracture which crosses the floor of the nose and lateral wall from the maxilla.

17 D. Such a condition is also associated with repeated chest infections and regurgitation of food. Management is typically surgical.

18 B. Smoking and alcohol are the most common risk factors in development of such a condition.

Extended matching questions

Theme: Neck swellings

1 E. Additional features include a lack of saliva production. Management is usually symptomatic.

2 H. Salivary gland malignancies are typically carcinomas and usually affect middle to older aged people.

3 C. Such tumours are highly vascular and hence their propensity to pulsate.

4 B. Management is typically surgical.

5 J. Such swellings are typically large and thick walled in nature. They may lead to stridor and cyanosis in certain cases.

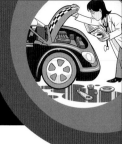

Single best answer

1 E.   A myocardial infarction is unlikely to be detected from a primary survey.

2 B.   Urethral damage is likely to be evident from a high riding prostate.

3 E.   Blood loss of 1500–2000 ml is indicative of type III haemorrhagic shock.

4 A.   A tension pneumothorax occurs when the pleura is breached allowing air to escape into the pleural cavity. Immediate management involves passing a large-bore IV cannula into the pleural cavity through the midclavicular line second intercostal space.

5 B.   An open pneumothorax allows air to be sucked into the pleural cavity on inspiration and forced out on expiration. Immediate management is to close the defect with occlusive dressing.

6 C.   A massive haemothorax is associated with the accumulation of over 1500 ml of blood in the chest. The chest is notably dull to percussion and breath sounds are absent.

7 D.   The fall has resulted in a flail chest. This occurs when one or more ribs are fractured in more than one place. The broken segment of chest wall moves independently from the rest of the chest resulting in a paradoxical motion. The underlying lung is often severely contused as a result.

8 B.   Cardiac tamponade is associated with a decrease in systolic pressure on inspiration, commonly known as pulsus paradoxus.

9 C.   When assessing such injuries one should bear in mind the components of AVPU (alertness, response to voice, response to pain and unresponsive) and GCS (eyes, voice and motor function) as a rule of thumb.

10 A.   Extradural haematomas are often associated with a head injury and are classically depicted by a brief period of unconsciousness followed by a lucid interval of recovery. A CT head is the gold standard investigation.

11 B.   Subdural haematomas are commonly seen in elderly, alcoholic individuals. These people are more susceptible on the background of their atrophic brains which make the connecting veins more likely to rupture.

12 D.   Classic hemisection of the spinal cord. A rare occurrence but resulting in ipsilateral power and proprioceptive loss below the lesion with contralateral loss of pain and temperature sensation.

13 A.   Burns are associated with severe fluid loss. This patient is in hypovolaemic shock and therefore the largest size cannula should be used namely 14G.

14 E.   For children under the age of 6 years an intraosseous needle in the proximal tibia is a useful emergency route for fluid administration in times of difficult access.

Extended matching questions

Theme: **Glasgow coma scale**

1 J.   Obeys commands = 6, normal speech = 5, spontaneous eye movement = 4.

2 A.   Flexes to pain = 3, incomprehensible sounds = 2, no eye movement = 1.

3 E.   Withdraws to pain = 4, confused speech = 4, eyes open to pain = 2.

4 D.   No motor response = 1, normal speech = 5, spontaneous eye movement = 4.

5 G.   Inappropriate speech = 3, obeys commands = 6, eyes opening on command = 3.

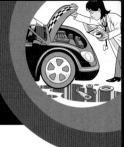

Single best answer

1 A. Urinalysis and culture are essential here. The patient has a urinary tract infection as noted by his urinary symptoms and associated pyrexia.

2 B. This is a severe urinary tract infection with associated pyrexia. Intravenous antibiotics such as cefuroxime or gentamicin may be of use.

3 D. Urinary symptoms and suprapubic tenderness are key features of acute cystitis.

4 B. Urinary symptoms with a sterile culture is diagnostic of interstitial cystitis.

5 C. Prostatitis manifests as urinary frequency and dysuria in addition to prostatic tenderness. It is commonly caused by *Escherichia coli* or *Staphylococcus aureus*.

6 E. Epididymo orchitis is commonly seen in young sexually active males. The offending organism is commonly *Chlamydia*.

7 D. Hypercalcaemia is a feature of renal cell carcinoma due to secretion of a parathormone like substance.

8 B. A CT scan is the most useful here in diagnosing a possible renal tumour.

9 D. The only curative treatment is a nephrectomy.

10 E. Most stones pass spontaneously. Stones greater than 5 mm require treatment.

11 A. This is a classic presentation of ureteric colic. Analgesia is of huge importance in helping to relieve the patient's symptoms.

12 A. The definitive investigation in bladder cancer. Biopsy will allow for staging assessment and ultimately choice of treatment.

13 A. This is a T2 tumour best treated with radical cystectomy.

14 A. Individuals with mild symptoms are best managed by watchful waiting as the risks of treatment usually outweigh the benefits.

15 B. An inguinal hernia is a common complication of undescended testes.

16 D. The patient has a seminoma. Lactate dehydrogenase and placental alkaline phosphatase are tumour markers of seminomas.

17 A. A classic description of a hydrocele.

18 B. Epididymo orchitis is commonly seen in young males and is particularly tender in nature.

19 C. A common presentation of an epididymal cyst.

20 E. Additional features would include swelling of the testicle and no relief of pain upon elevation of the scrotum. This is unlike epididymitis where elevation may help improve the pain.

Extended matching questions

Theme: Investigations

1 A. The diagnosis is a urinary tract infection most appropriately confirmed by a urine dipstick or urine microscopy and culture.

2 H. The diagnosis is renal colic. The clue is with regards to his long distance running and hence tendency to become severely dehydrated. An abdominal KUB is the most appropriate diagnostic tool.

3 D. The diagnosis is urinary tract obstruction specifically at the bladder. An ultrasound scan will help to detect evidence of obstruction and likely hydronephrosis.

4 C. The diagnosis is most probably prostatic carcinoma. Serum PSA is likely to be notably elevated.

5 G. The diagnosis is stress incontinence most appropriately diagnosed by urodynamic studies.

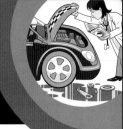

Single best answer

1 E.   Type I respiratory failure is due to failure of gas exchange despite adequate ventilation.

2 D.   Deficiencies in electrolytes such as potassium and phosphate are rare but known causes of respiratory failure. A low serum magnesium is not commonly associated with respiratory failure.

3 C.   This patient has notable features of sepsis, namely pyrexia, an elevated white cell count and C-reactive protein.

4 C.   Contrast used for radiological investigations/procedures is notorious for adversely affecting renal function as the contrast is nephrotoxic.

5 E.   According to current NICE (National Institute of Health and Clinical Excellence) guidelines none of the listed investigations are recommended prior to surgery.

6 B.   According to NICE, an ECG is highly recommended.

7 D.   According to NICE, a clotting screen is not essential prior to surgery.

8 E.   In this individual's case, NICE states lung function tests are not recommended.

9 A.   Bowel preparation in the form of Picolax or Kleen prep is recommended the day before surgery.

10 E.   According to the WHO (World Health Organisation) analgesic ladder, diclofenac would be the next recommended choice of drug.

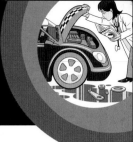
Single best answer

1 E. Renal calculi is a well recognised complication of ileostomy formation and not intrahepatic calculi.

2 C. Left-sided abdominal pain and dark red rectal bleeding are diagnostic features of ischaemic colitis.

3 B. This is the most definitive step in the treatment for sigmoid volvulus. Caecal volvulus requires immediate surgery.

4 D. Vitamin B12 deficiency anaemia is not a common feature of right-sided colonic tumours.

5 E. The diagnosis is haemorrhoids. Injection sclerotherapy is the preferred management option in such a condition with an overall success rate of up to 85%.

6 A. Classic presentation of a perianal haematoma. There is often a history of straining prior to the perianal pain.

7 D. Glyceryl trinitrate is regarded as the first-line form of management in those with an anal fissure. It helps to relax the internal anal sphincter, allowing fissure healing and thus relieving the pain.

8 C. Such studies help to measure internal and external sphincter pressures and assess integrity of the sphincter complex using endoanal ultrasound hence confirming such a diagnosis.

9 D. Classic presentation of an anal fistula.

10 B. The diagnosis is an oesophageal perforation in view of the presence of crepitus in the suprasternal notch. This is best investigated by a chest X-ray in the first instance.

11 A. The diagnosis is corrosive oesophagitis which involves an urgent endoscopy in the first instance to assess extent of damage.

12 E. Sliding hernias are associated with reflux disease and not rolling hernias.

13 C. The diagnosis is achalasia. The most effective management plan is Heller's myotomy which involves division of the muscles of the lower oesophageal sphincter.

14 C. This patient has evidence of jaundice. An abdominal ultrasound is of key importance in such cases in order to assess evidence of bile duct dilatation.

15 D. Malaria is an example of pre-hepatic jaundice. Malaria is associated with the breakdown of red blood cells and subsequent bilirubin production.

16 B. Jaundice is associated with decreased angiogenesis.

17 A. Hepatic haemangiomas are not amenable to biopsy as they are prone to bleeding.

18 E. The diagnosis most likely is liver cancer. Serum alpha fetoprotein is highly sensitive and specific for such cancers.

19 C. Gallstones are characteristically more common in females.

20 B. Antibiotics are not an important management step in biliary colic. They are more appropriately used in cholecystitis.

21 D. The diagnosis in this case is acute cholecystitis. Patients may often demonstrate Boas' sign which is hyperaesthesia below the right scapula.

22 B. The diagnosis is acute cholangitis in view of the triad of features, namely jaundice, abdominal pain and fever with associated rigors. *E. coli* is the most likely causative organism in such a presentation.

23 E. Secretin is released when gastric acid enters the duodenum.

24 C. A blood glucose concentration of greater than 10 mmol/l is an indicator of severity in acute pancreatitis.

25 C. Such tumour markers are notably elevated in pancreatic cancer.

26 B. Taking into account evidence of distant metastases the mainstay form of management would be palliative. Resection of such a tumour with the hope for cure is less than 15%.

27 A. Such a condition rarely causes splenomegaly.

28 A. This patient has developed overwhelming post splenectomy infection. In addition to preoperative immunisation, prophylactic therapy with penicillin V is highly recommended to reduce risk of infection from organisms such as *Haemophilus influenzae*, *Streptococcus pneumoniae* and meningococci.

29 D. Failure of medical management after a one month period is not an indication for surgery.

30 E. Ascites is rare occurring in less than 5% of cases.

31 C. The diagnosis is gastric cancer most appropriately investigated by endoscopy and biopsy.

32 B. Duke's stage B cancers extend into the muscularis or into or through the serosa. The latter is referred to as stage B2 and the former B1.

33 E. Malignancy is not a complication of acute diverticulitis.

Extended matching questions

Theme: Upper gastrointestinal disorders

1 D. Management typically involves the use of high-dose proton pump inhibitors or surgery.

2 G. Squamous cell carcinomas usually affect the middle third of the oesophagus and are due to a high intake of alcohol, smoking and salted fish consumption.

3 A. Chest X-ray features may show evidence of a fluid level behind the heart. Management typically involves surgical division of the lower oesophageal sphincter.

4 F. Characteristic features of a duodenal ulcer. Gastric ulcers typically result in pain after food.

5 I. Such swallowing difficulties are due to a web like formation in the upper part of the oesophagus.

Theme: Lower gastrointestinal disorders

1 B. Classic presentation of intussusception. Additional features may include a mass in the right iliac fossa. Management typically involves surgery.

2 C. Classic presentation of a peri anal haematoma.

3 F. In addition to colonoscopy a diagnosis of angiodysplasia is often made following arteriography.

4 E. Additional macroscopic features include the presence of skip lesions.

5 J. Complications include gangrene, perforation and stricture formation.

Theme: Hepatobiliary disorders

1 G. Classic presentation of biliary colic. The pain is often quite severe in nature and associated with episodes of vomiting.

2 D. Such tumours carry a poor prognosis with a 5 year survival rate of approximately 35% following surgery.

3 F. Such a finding is known as Boas' sign and is characteristic of acute cholecystitis.

4 A. This triad of features is known as Charcot's triad and is characteristic of cholangitis.

5 E. Other predisposing factors may include hepatitis or haemochromatosis. Treatment often involves surgical resection.

A

abdomen, acute, 75, 141
abdominal aortic aneurysm
    diagnosis, 79, 145
    features, 81–2, 145
    ruptured, 74, 79, 141, 145
abducens nerve palsy, 35, 125
absence seizure, 38, 126
absent pulses, 80, 145
acamprosate, 69, 137
acanthosis nigricans, 14, 116
acarbose, 25, 121
ACE inhibitors
    hyperkalaemia, 56, 133
    hypertension in diabetic patients, 58, 134
    renal failure, 27, 123
acetylcholine receptor antibodies, 33, 125
achalasia
    diagnosis, 61, 135
    dysphagia, 70, 138
    management, 106–7, 159
    signs, 110, 160
acoustic neuroma, 92, 151
acromegaly
    investigations, 17, 25, 119, 121
    presentation, 24, 120
acromioclavicular osteoarthritis, 87, 149
activated partial thromboplastin time (APTT), 46, 129
acute abdomen, 75, 141
acute coronary syndrome
    aspirin, 59, 134
    treatment, 56, 134
acute lymphoblastic leukaemia, 47, 129
acute myeloid leukaemia, 46, 129
acute nephritic syndrome, 31, 124
acute painful neuropathy, 24, 121
acute promyelocytic leukaemia, 46, 129
acute tubular necrosis, 27, 123
Addisonian crisis, 20, 119
Addison's disease, investigation, 20, 25, 119, 121
adenocarcinoma
    lung, 13, 116
    oesophagus, 61, 110, 135, 160
adenolymphoma, 91, 151
adenosine, supraventricular tachycardia, 133
adrenal gland insufficiency, 20, 119
adrenaline, anaphylactic reaction, 45, 129
adrenocorticotropic hormone (ACTH), Cushing's
        syndrome, 20, 120

agranulocytosis, 18, 119
airway obstruction, 95, 153
alanine aminotransferase (ALT)
    encephalopathy, 66, 136
    hepatitis B, 66, 136
albumin, nephrotic syndrome, 30, 123
alcohol, squamous cell carcinoma of the neck,
        93, 151
alcoholic cirrhosis, 67, 136
alcoholic liver disease, 68, 137
aldosterone to renin ratio, 22, 120
alginate, gastro oesophageal reflux disease, 69, 137
alkaline phosphatase, Paget's disease, 5, 113
allergic rhinitis, 93, 151
all-*trans* retinoic acid, 46, 129
alpha 1 antitrypsin deficiency, 69, 137
alpha blockers, benign prostatic hypertrophy,
        32, 124
alpha fetoprotein
    hepatocellular carcinoma, 68, 137
    liver cancer, 107, 159
    teratoma, 29, 123
amnesia, transient global, 39, 126
amoxicillin
    ear infection, 92, 151
    Helicobacter pylori treatment, 62, 135
    pneumonia, 11, 115
    urinary tract infection, 32, 124
amyloidosis, renal failure, 31, 124
anaemia
    of chronic disease, 49, 130
    colonoscopy, 63, 135
    haemolytic *see* haemolytic anaemia
    iron deficiency *see* iron deficiency anaemia
    macrocytic, 18, 49, 119, 130
    renal failure, 31, 124
    in rheumatoid arthritis, 3, 113
    treatment, 50, 130
    upper gastrointestinal endoscopy, 63, 135
anal fissure, 106, 159
anal fistula, 106, 159
analgesia
    post-operative, 104, 157
    renal colic, 29, 32, 123, 124
    sickle cell crisis, 50, 130
    ureteric colic, 100, 155
anaphylactic reaction, 45, 129
anaplastic thyroid carcinoma, 19, 119
anastrozole, 85, 147

aneurysm
  aortic *see* aortic aneurysm
  false, 80, 145
  mycotic, 80, 145
  popliteal artery, 80, 145
  posterior communicating artery, 40, 127
angina, 56, 58–9, 134
angiodysplasia
  diagnosis, 110, 160
  presentation, 69, 137
angiogenesis in jaundice, 107, 159
ankle brachial pressure index, 80, 145
ankylosing spondylitis
  back pain, 7, 114
  diagnosis, 4, 113
anorectal physiology studies, faecal incontinence,
    106, 159
antacids, gastro-oesophageal reflux disease, 69, 137
anterior cruciate ligament rupture, 88, 89, 149
antibiotics
  cholecystitis, 108, 159
  cystic fibrosis, 10, 115
  urinary tract infection, 99, 155
anti-centromere antibodies, systemic sclerosis, 4, 113
antihistamines, Meniere's disease, 92, 151
anti-La antibodies, Sjögren's syndrome, 5, 113
antimitochondrial antibodies (AMAs), primary biliary
    sclerosis, 67, 69, 136, 137
antinuclear antibodies
  autoimmune hepatitis, 66, 136
  discoid lupus, 4, 113
antiphospholipid syndrome, 6, 114
anti-Ro antibodies, Sjögren's syndrome, 5, 113
anti-thyroid stimulating hormone receptor antibodies,
    18, 119
aortic aneurysm
  abdominal *see* abdominal aortic aneurysm
  dissecting, 75, 81–2, 141, 145
  thoracic, 79, 145
aortic dissection, 58–9, 134
aortic regurgitation, 55, 133
aortic stenosis
  clinical features, 59, 134
  signs, 54, 133
aplastic anaemia, 50, 130
appendicitis diagnosis, 73, 141
arterial blood gases *see* blood gases (arterial)
arterial leg ulcers, 81, 145
arteriography, angiodysplasia, 160
artery of Adamkiewicz, 79, 145
arthritis, 6, 114
  osteoarthritis *see* osteoarthritis
  psoriatic 4, 6, 113, 114
  reactive, 4, 6, 113, 114
  rheumatoid, 3, 6, 113, 114
asbestos-induced lung damage, 12, 116

ascites, 74, 141
  gastric cancer, 109, 160
  hepatocellular carcinoma, 68, 137
  Meig's syndrome, 67, 136
aspartate aminotransferase (AST), hepatitis B,
    66, 136
aspirin
  acute coronary syndrome, 59, 134
  cerebral infarct, 40, 126
  myocardial infarction, 57, 134
  stroke, 69, 137
asthma, 10, 115
ataxic gait, 41, 127
atrial fibrillation, 54, 74, 133, 141
atrial flutter, 53, 54, 133
Auer rods, 46, 129
auranofin, 7, 114
autoimmune haemolytic anaemia, 50, 130
autoimmune hepatitis, 136
autoimmune thrombocytopenic purpura, 45, 129
autonomic neuropathy, 31, 124

B
Bacillus cereus, 70, 138
background retinopathy, 24, 121
back pain
  causes of, 7, 114
  low, 80, 145
bacterial meningitis, 36, 125
bacterial peritonitis, 67, 136
beak deformity, oesophageal, 61, 135
Behcet's disease, 6, 114
benign essential tremor, 37, 126
benign oesophageal stricture, 70, 138
benign prostatic hyperplasia, 100, 155
benign prostatic hypertrophy, 32, 124
beta blockers, atrial fibrillation, 54, 133
beta human chorionic gonadotrophin, teratoma,
    29, 123
beta thalassaemia major, 50, 130
bilateral diffuse pleural thickening, 12, 116
biliary colic, 108, 110, 159, 160
biochemistry, normal values, x
biopsy
  bladder cancer, 100, 155
  gastric cancer, 109, 160
  liver tumours, 107, 159
bisoprolol, atrial fibrillation, 54, 133
bisphosphonates, osteoporosis, 5, 113
bitemporal hemianopia, 17, 119
bladder cancer
  investigations, 100, 155
  treatment, 100, 155
blood cultures
  Hickman line, 65, 136
  infective endocarditis, 57, 134

blood gases (arterial)
  acute pancreatitis, 73, 141
  chronic obstructive pulmonary disease (COPD),
    9, 115
  normal values, x
blood glucose
  acute pancreatitis, 108, 159
  epilepsy, 39, 126
blood loss, 95, 153
blood pressure control, 30, 124
Boas' sign, 108, 110, 159, 160
botulin toxin, dystonia, 37, 126
Boutonniere deformity, 114
bowel obstruction, 75, 141
bowel preparation, 104, 157
branchial cyst, 91, 151
branchial sinus, 93, 151
BRCA1/BRCA2, 83–4, 147
breast cancer
  chemotherapy, 84–5, 147
  ductal, 84, 147
  family history, 83–4, 147
  management, 85, 147
  risk factors, 83, 147
  screening, 84, 147
  staging, 84, 147
  survival rate, 84, 147
breast cysts, 83, 84, 147
breast disease, 83–5, 147
breast lumps, 83–4, 103–4, 147, 157
bronchiectasis, 9, 15, 115, 117
bronchitis, 15, 117
Brown Sequard syndrome, 96, 153
Buerger's disease, 81–2, 145
Burkitt's lymphoma, 48, 129
burns, 97, 153

C

CA 19–9, pancreatic cancer, 108, 159
calcium, renal failure, 28, 123
callus formation, 89, 149
Campylobacter, 70, 138
Candida infection, 70, 138
captopril, 59, 134
carbamazepine, epilepsy, 42, 127
carbimazole, exophthalmus, 18, 119
carcinoembryonic antigen (CEA), pancreatic cancer,
  108, 159
cardiac murmurs investigation, 55, 133
cardiac syndrome X, 56, 134
cardiac tamponade, 95, 96, 153
cardiomyopathy
  dilated, 58, 134
  hypertrophic, 58, 134
cardiovascular medicine, 53–9, 133–4
carina, narrowed, 55, 133

carotid body tumour, 91, 93, 151
carotid sinus massage, 54, 133
carpal tunnel syndrome, 41–2, 127
carpometacarpal joint, first, 3, 113
catecholamines, phaeochromocytoma, 22, 120
cauda equina syndrome
  back pain, 7, 114
  investigation, 88, 149
cefotaxime, meningococcal septicaemia, 36, 125
cefuroxime, urinary tract infections, 30, 99, 123
cerebral hemisphere infarct, 39, 126
cerebral infarct, 40, 126
cerebrospinal fluid (CSF)
  meningitis, 36, 125
  multiple sclerosis, 36, 126
  subarachnoid haemorrhage, 39, 126
Charcot Marie Tooth disease, 41–2, 127
Charcot's triad, 110, 160
chemotherapy
  breast cancer, 84–5, 147
  colon cancer, 65, 136
  seminoma, 29, 123
cherry red spot, macular, 35, 125
chest injury, 95–6, 153
chest pain, 58–9, 134
chest X-ray
  achalasia, 160
  cryptogenic fibrosing alveolitis, 15, 117
  oesophageal perforation, 106, 159
  pneumonia, 11, 115
Child's grading, 136
Chlamydia psittaci, pneumonia, 11, 14, 115, 116
Chlamydia spp., epididymo-orchitis, 155
cholangiocarcinoma, 110, 160
cholangitis
  acute, 108, 159
  Charcot's triad, 110, 160
cholecystitis
  acute, 108, 159
  antibiotics, 108, 159
  Boas' sign, 110, 160
  diagnosis, 75, 141
  investigation, 68, 137
chorea, levodopa, 37, 126
chronic lymphocytic leukaemia, 47, 129
chronic myeloid leukaemia, 47, 129
chronic obstructive pulmonary disease (COPD), 9,
  15, 115, 117
ciclosporin, colitis, 64, 136
cirrhosis
  alcoholic, 67, 136
  primary biliary, 67, 69, 136, 137
  prothrombin time, 66, 136
clarithromycin, Helicobacter pylori, 62, 135
clotting process, 45, 129
clotting screen, preoperative, 104, 157

cluster headache, 34, 125
coagulation, normal values, x
coeliac disease
    anaemia, 49, 130
    diagnosis, 63, 135
    features, 63, 135
    investigation, 63, 135
cold antibody haemolysis, 50, 130
cold exposure, 50, 130
colitis
    ischaemic, 105, 110, 159, 160
    steroids, 64, 136
    ulcerative see ulcerative colitis
colloids, pulseless electrical activity, 54, 133
colon cancer, 64, 136
    Duke's B, 64–5, 136
    Duke's C, 65, 136
    family history, 65, 136
    features, 105, 159
    staging, 64–5, 109, 136, 160
    treatment, 65, 136
colonoscopy
    anaemia, 63, 135
    angiodysplasia, 160
    coeliac disease, 63, 135
compartment syndrome, 90, 150
complete heart block, 53, 133
complex partial seizure, 38, 126
compression stockings
    lymphoedema, 81, 145
    varicose veins, 81, 145
computed tomography (CT)
    acute diverticulitis, 64, 136
    bronchiectasis, 9, 115
    pancreatitis, 68, 73, 137, 141
    renal tumours, 100, 155
    stroke, 40, 126
    subarachnoid haemorrhage, 39, 126
computed tomography pulmonary angiogram (CTPA),
        pulmonary embolism, 14, 116
Congo Red staining, amyloidosis, 31, 124
connective tissue disease, 6, 114
constipation, 64, 136
Coomb's test, 50, 130
corrosive oesophagitis, 106, 159
corticosteroids, acute pericarditis, 134
costochondritis, 58–9, 134
cotton wool exudates, 134
cough, captopril, 59, 134
cranial nerve lesions, 41, 81, 127, 145
    see also specific cranial nerve
creatinine, 28, 123
Crohn's disease
    features, 110, 160
    ileoscopy, 65, 136
    risk factors, 63, 135

Crohn's disease (continued)
    steroids, 64, 136
    treatment, 64, 69, 136, 137
cryptogenic fibrosing alveolitis, 12, 15, 116, 117
Cullen's sign, 74, 141
Cushing's syndrome
    causes, 20, 120
    features, 13, 116
    investigation, 25, 121
    lymphocytes, 19, 119
    treatment, 21
cyclophosphamide, 85, 147
cystectomy, bladder cancer, 100, 155
cystic fibrosis
    bronchiectasis, 15, 117
    diagnosis, 9, 115
    management, 10, 115
cystic hygroma, 93, 151
cystitis
    acute, 99, 155
    interstitial, 99, 155
cystometrogram
    overflow incontinence, 29, 123
    stress incontinence, 32, 101–2, 124, 155
cystoscopy, bladder cancer, 100, 155
cytomegalovirus, 51, 130

D
daytime sleepiness, 9, 115
deep vein thrombosis (DVT), 46, 129
de Quervain's thyroiditis, 24, 120
dermatomyositis, 4, 62, 113, 135
developmental dysplasia of the hip, 89, 149
dexamethasone suppression test, 25, 121
dextrose, hypoglycaemia, 23, 120
diabetes insipidus
    diagnosis, 21, 120
    investigation, 25, 121
diabetes mellitus
    complications, 24, 121
    hypoglycaemia, 23, 120
    in pregnancy, 23, 120
    type 2, 22, 120
diabetic amyotrophy, 24, 121
diabetic ketoacidosis, 23, 120
dialysis, 27, 28, 123
diaphragmatic hernia, 78, 143
diarrhoea, metformin, 22, 120
diazepam, epilepsy, 38, 126
diclofenac
    peptic ulcer, 62, 135
    post-operative analgesia, 104, 157
diet therapy, diabetes mellitus, 22, 120
diffuse oesophageal spasm, 61, 135
dilated cardiomyopathy, 58, 134
direct inguinal hernia, 77, 143

discoid lupus, 4, 6, 113, 114
disease-modifying antirheumatic drugs (DMARDs), 3, 113
dissecting aortic aneurysm, 75, 81–2, 141, 145
diuretics
    alcoholic cirrhosis, 67, 136
    heart failure, 56, 133
    hypertension in diabetic patients, 58, 134
diverticulitis
    acute, 64, 109, 136, 160
    investigation, 74, 141
dopamine, Parkinson's disease, 37, 126
Doppler ultrasound
    deep vein thrombosis, 46, 129
    sapheno-femoral competence, 81, 145
drip and suck technique, 73, 141
drug(s)
    cardiovascular medicine, 59, 134
    diabetes, 25, 121
    endocrinology, 25, 121
    gastroenterology and hepatobiliary medicine, 69, 137
    respiratory disease, 14, 116
    rheumatology, 7, 114
    see also specific drug
Duchenne muscular dystrophy, 33, 42, 125, 127
ductal breast cancer, 84, 147
duct papilloma, 83, 147
duodenal ulcer, 69, 110, 137, 160
Dupuytren's contracture, 88, 149
dysphagia, 70, 138
dystonia, 37, 126
dystrophia myotonica, 42, 127

E

ear, nose and throat, 91–3, 151
ear infection, 92, 151
Eaton Lambert syndrome, 14, 116
echocardiography (ECHO)
    cardiac murmurs, 55, 133
    heart failure, 55, 133
    pericardial effusion, 58, 134
eighth cranial nerve, 41, 127
electrical cardioversion, 54, 133
electrocardiogram (ECG), preoperative, 104, 157
electrolytes, renal failure, 27, 123
embolectomy, 74, 141
emphysema, 15, 116
empty sella syndrome, 24, 120
encephalopathy
    grade 3, 66, 136
    hepatic, 67, 136
endocarditis, 57, 134
    infective see infective endocarditis
endocrinology, 17–25, 119–21
endoscopy
    corrosive oesophagitis, 106, 159
    gastric cancer, 109, 160

enoxaparin, 56, 134
epididymal cyst, 101, 155
epididymitis, 75, 141
epididymo-orchitis, 99, 101, 155
epigastric hernia, 77, 143
epilepsy, 37–9, 42, 126, 127
Epstein-Barr virus, 51, 130
ergotamine, headache, 125
erythropoietin, anaemia, 31, 124
Escherichia coli
    acute cholangitis, 108, 159
    bacterial peritonitis, 67, 136
    gastroenteritis, 70, 138
    prostatitis, 155
    urinary tract infection, 30, 123
ethambutol, 14, 116
ethosuximide, side effects, 38, 126
exophthalmus, 18, 19, 119
external beam radiotherapy, 28–9, 123
extradural haematoma, 96, 153
extradural haemorrhage, 39, 126
extrapyramidal diseases, 42–3, 127
extrinsic allergic alveolitis
    causes, 12, 116
    X-ray features, 15, 117
eye(s), sarcoidosis, 12, 116

F

facial nerve, 41, 127
factor V abnormalities, 46, 129
factor VII, clotting, 45, 129
factor VIII, haemophilia A, 45, 129
faecal incontinence, 106, 159
false aneurysm, 80, 145
family history, colon cancer, 65, 136
farmer's lung, 12, 116
fat embolism, 90, 149
femoral hernia, 77, 143
femur fracture, intracapsular neck of, 90, 149
ferritin, haemochromatosis, 68, 136–7
fibroadenoma, breast, 83, 147
fibroadenosis, 83, 147
fifth cranial nerve, 41, 127
fine-needle aspiration cytology, goitre, 19, 119
finger clubbing
    cryptogenic fibrosing alveolitis, 12, 116
    cystic fibrosis, 9, 115
    lung cancer, 13, 116
first degree AV block, 53, 133
fistula in ano, 106, 159
flail chest, 95, 96, 153
flexible sigmoidoscopy, 105, 159
flucloxacillin
    pneumonia, 14, 116
    Staphylococcus aureus, 4, 113

fluid replacement, intravenous *see* intravenous fluid replacement
fluid restriction, syndrome of inappropriate antidiuretic hormone (SIADH), 21, 120
focal motor seizure, 38, 126
folate
  deficiency, 126
  replacement, 49, 130
folic acid, ischaemic heart disease, 56, 134
follicle stimulating hormone (FSH), 17, 119
fourth cranial nerve, 41, 127
fractures, 90, 149
  callus formation, 89, 149
  complications, 90, 149–50
  Le Fort classification system, 93, 151
  osteoarthritis, 89, 149
Friedrich's ataxia, 34, 125
frontal lobe tumours, 35, 125
fucidin, 4, 113
furosemide, pulmonary oedema, 56, 133

G
galactorrhoea, 17, 119
gall bladder
  calculi, 64, 135
  disease, 74, 141
gallstones, 107, 159
gastric cancer
  investigations, 109, 160
  signs, 109, 160
  upper gastrointestinal endoscopy, 62, 135
gastric ulcer, 160
gastroenteritis, 70, 138
gastroenterology, 61–70, 135–8
gastrointestinal bleeding, 67, 69, 136, 137
gastrointestinal disorders, 110, 160
gastrointestinal surgery, 105–10, 159–60
gastrointestinal tract, non-Hodgkin's lymphoma, 48, 129
gastro-oesophageal reflux disease
  diagnosis, 59, 135
  treatment, 61, 69, 135, 137
Gaucher's disease, 51, 131
gentamicin
  toxicity, 127
  urinary tract infection, 30, 99, 123
giant-cell arteritis, 34, 35, 125
Glasgow Coma Scale (GCS), 40, 97, 126, 153
glibenclamide, 25, 121
glomerulonephritis, 30, 123, 136
glucose–6-phosphate dehydrogenase deficiency, 50, 130
glue ear, 92, 151
glyceryl trinitrate (GTN)
  anal fissure, 106, 159
  angina, 56, 134
goitre, 19, 119
gout, 5, 113

grand mal seizures, 42, 127
Graves' disease, 18, 24, 119, 120
Guillain-Barré syndrome, 33, 41–2, 125, 127

H
haematology, 45–51, 129–31
  normal values, x
haematuria, 30, 124
haemochromatosis
  diagnosis, 68, 136–7
  features, 69, 137
  investigations, 5, 113
  management, 69
  treatment, 137
haemolytic anaemia, 49, 130
  autoimmune, 50, 130
  warm antibody, 50, 130
haemophilia A, 45, 129
Haemophilus influenzae
  otitis media, 92, 151
  pneumonia, 14, 116
haemorrhagic shock, 95, 153
haemorrhoids
  management, 69, 105, 137, 159
  symptoms, 69, 137
hands
  osteoarthritis, 3
  pain, 3, 4, 113
Hashimoto's thyroiditis, 17, 24, 119, 121
headache
  cluster, 34, 125
  management, 35, 125
  severity, 96, 153
head injury, 96, 153
heart block
  complete, 53, 133
  first degree AV, 53, 133
  Mobitz type 1, 53, 133
  Mobitz type 2, 53, 133
heartburn, 61, 135
heart disease
  clinical features, 59, 134
  see also specific disease
heart failure
  captopril, 59, 134
  diuretics, 56, 133
  echocardiography (ECHO), 55, 133
Heberden's nodes, 114
Helicobacter pylori
  mechanisms, 61, 135
  treatment, 62, 135
Heller's myotomy, 106–7, 159
hemiballismus, 42–3, 127
Henoch-Schonlein purpura, 5, 113
heparin, unfractioned, 46, 129
hepatic encephalopathy, 67, 136

hepatic haemangiomas, 107, 159
hepatitis, autoimmune, 136
hepatitis A, 66, 136
hepatitis B, 66, 136
hepatitis C, 66, 136
hepatobiliary disorders, 69, 110,
     137, 160
hepatobiliary medicine, 61–70, 135–8
hepatocellular carcinoma, 68, 137
hepatoma, 110, 160
herceptin, 85, 147
hereditary elliptocytosis, 50, 130
hereditary spherocytosis, 50, 130
hernia, 77–8, 143
     see also specific type
hiatus hernia, 106, 159
Hickman line, blood cultures, 65, 136
hip dislocation, 89, 149
HIV virus, 51, 130
Hodgkin's disease, 47–8, 129
homonymous quadrantanopia, 40, 127
horizontal fissure, 55, 133
Horner's syndrome, 14, 116
humeral shaft fracture, 90, 149
Huntington's disease, 42–3, 127
hydrocele, 101, 155
hydrocortisone
     Addisonian crisis, 20, 119
     hypothyroidism, 18, 119
hydrogen breath test, 63, 135
hydroxychloroquine, 7, 114
hyperaldosteronism, 22, 120
hypercalcaemia
     leukaemia, 21, 120
     renal cell carcinoma, 99, 155
hyperglycaemia, 68, 137
hyperkalaemia
     ACE inhibitors, 56, 133
     bowel motility, 64, 136
hyperparathyroidism, 21, 120
hyperprolactinaemia, 17, 119
hypertension
     control, 80, 145
     diabetic patients, 58, 134
     retinal disease, 58, 134
hyperthyroidism, 18, 119
hypertrophic cardiomyopathy, 58, 134
hypertrophic pulmonary osteoarthropathy,
     14, 116
hypoadrenalism, 20, 119
hypocalcaemia, 21, 120
hypoglossal (XII) nerve, 81, 145
hypoglycaemia, 23, 120
hyponatraemia, 46, 129
hypopituitarism, 17, 119
hypothyroidism, 18, 119

ileoscopy, Crohn's disease, 65, 136
ileostomy, 105, 159
imatinib, 47, 129
incisional hernia, 77–8, 143
indigestion, 69, 137
indirect inguinal hernia, 77, 143
infective endocarditis
     clinical features, 59, 134
     Staphylococcus aureus, 57, 134
inflammatory bowel disease, 63, 64, 135
influenza, 15, 116
inguinal hernia, 78, 143
     direct, 77, 143
     indirect, 77, 143
injection sclerotherapy, haemorrhoids, 105, 159
insulin, diabetes mellitus, 22, 120
intermittent claudication, 80, 145
internal carotid artery bruit, 40, 126
International Normalised Ratio (INR), 46, 129
International Prostate Symptom Score, 100, 155
interphalangeal joints
     distal, 3, 4, 113
     proximal, 3, 113
interstitial cystitis, 99, 155
intervertebral discs, prolapsed, 7, 114
intravenous fluid replacement
     distended loops of small bowel, 73, 141
     hypercalcaemia, 21, 120
     melaena, 62, 135
     thyroid crisis, 19, 119
intravenous urogram, renal colic, 74, 141
intrinsic factor autoantibodies, 49, 130
intussusception, 110, 160
investigations
     diabetes, 25, 121
     endocrinology, 25, 121
     renal medicine, 32, 124
     respiratory medicine, 15, 117
     see also specific disease; specific investigation
iron deficiency anaemia
     investigations, 63, 135
     menstruation, 49, 130
ischaemic colitis, 105, 110, 159, 160
ischaemic heart disease
     heart failure, 55, 133
     risk factors, 56, 134
isoniazid, 41–2, 127

Jacksonian motor seizure, 38, 42, 126, 127
jaundice
     pre-hepatic, 107, 159
     ultrasonography, 65, 107, 136, 159
joint fluid microscopy, pseudogout, 5, 113

K

Kala azar, 51, 131
Kallman's syndrome, 24, 120
kidneys, ureters and bladder (KUB) X-ray
    renal colic, 101, 155
    renal stones, 29–30, 123
knees
    pain and stiffness, 3, 4, 113
    swelling, 113
Kuchitsky cells, 116

L

lactate dehydrogenase, seminoma, 101, 155
lactic acidosis, 22, 120
lactic dehydrogenase levels, pleural effusion, 13
laryngotracheobronchitis, 15, 117
lateral epicondylitis, 88, 149
lateral medullary syndrome, 40, 126
Le Fort classification system, 93, 151
Legionella pneumophila, 14, 116
legionellosis, 11, 115
leukaemia
    acute lymphoblastic, 47, 129
    acute myeloid, 46, 129
    acute promyelocytic, 46, 129
    chronic lymphocytic, 47, 129
    chronic myeloid, 47, 129
    lymphadenopathy, 51, 130
levodopa, chorea, 37, 126
limb girdle dystrophy, 42, 127
lipids, normal values, x
lipoproteins, normal values, x
lithium, 21, 120
liver cancer, alpha fetoprotein, 107, 159
liver function tests, 66, 136
liver tumours biopsy, 107, 159
lower gastrointestinal disorders, 110, 160
lower limb ischaemia, 74, 80, 141, 145
lumbar puncture, meningitis, 36, 125
lung cancer, 14–15, 116
    adenocarcinoma, 13, 116
    small cell, 13, 116
    smoking, 13, 116
    squamous cell, 13, 116
lung function tests, 104, 157
luteinizing hormone (LH), hypopituitarism, 17, 119
lymphadenopathy, 51, 130
    sarcoidosis, 12, 116
lymph node biopsy
    Hodgkin's disease, 47, 129
    sarcoidosis, 12, 116
lymphocytes, Cushing's syndrome, 19, 119
lymphoedema, 81, 145
lymphoma, 51, 130
    see also Hodgkin's disease; non-Hodgkin's
      lymphoma

M

McBurney's point, 73, 141
macrocytic anaemia, 18, 49, 119, 130
macrocytosis, 49, 130
macrophages, tuberculosis, 11, 115
magnesium, low serum, 103, 157
magnetic resonance angiography, renal artery stenosis, 32, 124
magnetic resonance imaging (MRI)
    cauda equina syndrome, 88, 149
    multiple sclerosis, 36, 125
    osteomyelitis, 87, 149
    syringomyelia, 34, 125
malaria, 51, 107, 131, 159
mallory bodies, 68, 137
Mallory Weiss tear, 62, 69, 135, 137
MALT lymphoma, 48, 129
malunion, fractures, 90, 150
mammary ducts ectasia, 83, 147
mammography, 84, 147
massive pneumothorax, 96, 153
M bands, 130
median nerve damage, 33, 125
medullary cell thyroid cancer, 19, 119
medullary spongy kidney, 31, 124
Meig's syndrome, 67, 136
melaena, 62, 135
Meniere's disease, 92, 151
meningitis
    bacterial, 36, 125
    investigation, 36, 125
    Streptococcus pneumoniae, 36, 125
meningococcal septicaemia, 36, 125
menstruation, iron deficiency anaemia, 49, 130
mesalazine, Crohn's disease, 69, 137
metanephrines, phaeochromocytoma, 22, 25, 120, 121
metatarsophalangeal joint, first, 6, 114
metformin
    diabetes mellitus, 22, 120
    side effects, 25, 121
    uses, 25, 121
methotrexate, rheumatoid arthritis, 3, 113
metronidazole
    Helicobacter pylori treatment, 62, 135
    pneumonia, 14, 116
microscopic polyangiitis, 6, 114
micturition problems, 4, 113
middle cerebral artery occlusion, 39, 126
middle meningeal artery rupture, 39, 126
migraine, 35, 125
mitral regurgitation, 54, 59, 133, 134
mitral stenosis, 54, 55, 133
Mobitz type 1 block, 53, 133
Mobitz type 2 block, 53, 133
motor neurone disease, 34, 125
multiple myeloma, 48, 129

multiple sclerosis
   ataxic gait, 41, 127
   cerebrospinal fluid, 36, 125
   presentation, 42–3, 127
murmurs investigation, 55, 133
muscle biopsy, poliomyositis, 4, 113
muscle diseases, 42, 127
muscle pains, 5, 113
myasthenia gravis, 33, 42, 125, 127
Mycobacterium tuberculosis, 11, 115
Mycoplasma pneumoniae, 11, 115
mycotic aneurysm, 80, 145
myelofibrosis, 45, 129
myeloma, 34, 125
   multiple, 48, 129
myocardial infarction
   aspirin, 57, 134
   diagnosis, 95, 153
   features, 58–9, 134
   pericarditis, 57, 134
   posterior, 57, 134
   troponin, 57, 134
myoclonus, 37, 126
myotonia, 33, 125
myotonia congenita, 42, 127

N

nail pitting, 4, 113
nasogastric decompression, 73, 141
neck
   squamous cell carcinoma of the, 93, 151
   swellings, 93, 151
nephrectomy, renal cell carcinoma, 100, 155
nephritic syndrome, acute, 31, 124
nephrotic syndrome
   causes, 30, 123
   clinical features, 31, 124
   management, 31, 124
   prednisolone, 32, 124
neurology, 33–43, 125–7
neuropathic ulcers, 80, 145
neuropathy
   acute painful, 24, 121
   autonomic, 31, 124
nifedipine, 59, 134
night sweats, Hodgkin's disease, 48, 129
night terrors, 38, 126
non-Hodgkin's lymphoma, 48, 129
non-steroidal anti-inflammatory drugs
     (NSAIDs)
   acute pericarditis, 134
   gout, 5, 113
   osteoarthritis, 3, 113
   tennis elbow, 88, 149
non-union, fractures, 90, 150
normal values, x

nosebleed, 92, 151
nystagmus, multiple sclerosis, 41, 127

O

obesity, metformin, 22, 120
obstructive sleep apnoea, 9, 115
obturator hernia, 78, 143
occupational respiratory disease, 10, 12, 115, 116
oculomotor nerve palsy, 35, 40, 41, 125, 127
oedema, sodium restricted diet, 30, 123
oesophageal web, 70, 138
oesophagitis, corrosive, 106, 159
oesophagus
   adenocarcinoma, 110, 160
   cork screw appearance, 61, 135
   diffuse spasm, 61, 135
   perforation, 106, 159
   squamous cell carcinoma, 61, 135
   stricture, benign, 70, 138
oligoclonal bands, 36, 126
omeprazole
   Helicobacter pylori treatment, 62, 135
   indigestion, 69, 137
open pneumothorax, 95, 153
ophthalmoplegia
   Graves' disease, 18, 119
   management, 19, 119
optic nerve, 41, 126, 127
oral glucose tolerance test, 17, 25, 119, 121
orthopaedics, 87–90, 149–50
osteoarthritis
   acromioclavicular, 87, 149
   affected joints, 3, 113
   features, 6, 114
   fractures, 89, 149
osteomalacia, 5, 113
   phenytoin side effects, 126
   renal failure, 31, 124
osteomyelitis, 87, 149
osteoporosis, 5, 113
osteosarcoma, 87, 149
osteosclerosis, renal failure, 31, 124
otitis externa, 92, 151
otitis media, 92, 151
overflow incontinence, 29, 123
oxygen therapy, 9, 115

P

Paget's disease
   bone, 5, 113
   nipple, 85, 147
palliative treatment, pancreatic cancer, 68, 108,
     137, 159
Pancoast's tumour, 14, 116
pancreatic cancer
   management, 23, 68, 120, 137

pancreatic cancer *(continued)*
   palliative treatment, 68, 108, 137, 159
   tumour markers, 108, 159
pancreatic function, 108, 159
pancreatitis
   acute, 68, 73, 108, 137, 141, 159
   chronic, 68, 137
   features, 75, 141
pantaloon hernia, 78, 143
paracetamol, osteoarthritis, 3, 113
parkinsonism plus, 37, 42–3, 126, 127
Parkinson's disease, 37, 126
parotitis, 91, 151
paroxysmal nocturnal haemoglobinuria, 50, 130
peak expiratory flow rate (PEFR), asthma, 10, 115
penicillamine, 7, 114
penicillin V, 109, 160
peptic ulcer
   causes, 62, 135
   indications for surgery, 109, 160
   symptoms, 62, 135
perforated viscus, 75, 141
perianal haematoma
   diagnosis, 106, 159
   presentation, 110, 160
pericardial effusion, 58, 134
pericarditis
   acute, 58, 134
   chest pain, 58–9, 134
   myocardial infarction, 57, 134
perinuclear anti-neutrophil cytoplasmic antibodies
   (pANCA), 6, 114
perioperative care, 103–4, 157
peripheral nerve diseases, 41–2, 127
peritoneal dialysis, 28, 123
peritonitis
   bacterial, 67, 136
   peritoneal dialysis, 28, 123
Perthes' disease, 89, 149
petit mal seizure, 38, 42, 126, 127
phaeochromocytoma
   investigation, 25, 121
   presentation, 22, 120
pharyngeal pouch, 70, 93, 138, 151
phenytoin
   epilepsy, 42, 127
   side effects, 38, 126
Philadelphia chromosome, 47, 129, 130
phosphate
   low serum, 103, 157
   renal failure, 28, 123
phosphate enema, 104, 157
phylloides tumour, 85, 147
pituitary adenoma, 20, 21, 120
pituitary apoplexy, 24, 120
pituitary disease, 24, 120

pituitary tumours, 17, 24, 119, 120
pizotifen, headache, 35, 125
plasma osmolality, diabetes insipidus, 25, 121
platelets, autoimmune thrombocytopenic purpura, 45, 129
pleomorphic adenoma, 91, 151
pleural effusion, 13, 116
pleural fluid, 13, 116
pleural thickening, bilateral diffuse, 12, 116
Plummer Vinson syndrome, 70, 110, 138, 160
pneumonia, 14, 116
   fracture complications, 90, 149
   investigations, 15, 117
   risk factors, 10, 115
   Streptococcus pneumoniae, 10, 115
pneumothorax
   massive, 96, 153
   open, 95, 153
   tension, 95, 153
poliomyelitis, 4, 113
poliomyositis, 6, 114
polyarteritis nodosa, 6, 114
polycystic kidney disease (PKD)
   adult-onset, 28, 123
   features, 31, 124
   investigation, 28, 123
polycythaemia vera, 45, 129
polymyalgia, 6, 114
popliteal artery aneurysm, 80, 145
posterior communicating artery, berry aneurysm, 40, 127
posterior cruciate ligament rupture, 89, 149
posterior inferior cerebellar artery, 40, 126
potassium
   high, 27, 123
   low serum, 103, 157
PR bleed, 62, 135
prednisolone
   asthma, 10, 115
   nephrotic syndrome, 32, 124
pregnancy, diabetes mellitus in, 23, 120
pre-proliferative retinopathy, 23, 24, 120, 121
primary biliary cirrhosis, 67, 69, 136, 137
primary sclerosing cholangitis, 69, 137
prolactin, galactorrhoea, 17, 119
propranolol
   contraindications, 59, 134
   exophthalmus, 18, 119
prostate gland, high/low riding, 95, 153
prostate specific antigen (PSA), 28, 101–2, 123, 155
prostatic cancer, 28–9, 101–2, 123, 155
prostatitis, 99, 155
protein
   Guillain-Barré syndrome, 33, 125
   nephrotic syndrome, 30, 123
   pleural effusion, 13

protein electrophoresis, multiple myeloma, 48, 130
prothrombin time, liver function in cirrhosis, 66, 136
proton pump inhibitors
    gastro-oesophageal reflux disease, 69, 137
    heartburn, 61, 135
    Helicobacter pylori treatment, 62, 135
    Zollinger-Ellison syndrome, 160
pseudobulbar palsy, 41, 127
pseudogout, 5, 113
Pseudomonas aeruginosa, 14, 116
psoriatic arthritis, 4, 6, 113, 114
pulmonary embolism, 14, 116
pulmonary hypertension, 59, 134
pulmonary oedema, furosemide, 56, 133
pulseless electrical activity, 54, 133
pulses, absent, 80, 145
pyrazinamide, 14, 116

R

radial nerve injury, 88, 149
radical cystectomy, bladder cancer, 100, 155
radical nephrectomy, renal cell carcinoma,
    100, 155
radioactive iodine, 18, 19, 119
radiological contrast, nephrotoxicity, 103, 157
radius fracture, distal, 90, 149
Ramsay Hunt syndrome, 41, 127
rash
    discoid lupus, 4, 113
    Henoch-Schonlein purpura, 5, 113
    peri-orbital, 62, 135
Raynaud's disease, 81–2, 145
reactive arthritis, 4, 6, 113, 114
rectal bleeding, 62, 135
rectal examination, 62, 135
red cells
    cigar-shaped, 50, 130
    tear drop shaped, 45, 129
reflux oesophagitis, 69, 137
renal artery stenosis, 32, 59, 124, 134
renal carcinoma, clinical features, 31, 124
renal cell carcinoma
    hypercalcaemia, 99, 155
    surgery, 28, 32, 123, 124
    treatment, 100, 155
renal colic
    analgesia, 29, 32, 123, 124
    diagnosis, 74, 141
    investigations, 32, 124
    kidneys, ureters and bladder (KUB) X-ray,
        101, 155
    presentation, 75, 141
renal disease, 31, 124
    clinical features, 31, 124
    management, 32, 124
    see also specific disease

renal failure, 22, 120
    acute, 28, 123
    acute tubular necrosis, 27, 123
    chronic, 28, 31, 123, 124
    complications, 31, 124
    dialysis, 27, 123
    investigation, 27, 28, 123
renal medicine, 27–32, 123–4
renal osteodystrophy, 27, 123
renal stones
    clinical features, 31, 124
    ileostomy complications, 105, 159
    investigation, 29–30, 123
renal tumours, 100, 155
repaglinide, 25, 121
respiratory failure, perioperative, 103, 157
respiratory medicine, 9–15, 115–17
respiratory tract diseases, 15, 116–17
reticulocyte count, haemolytic anaemia, 49, 130
retinal disease, grade 3, 58, 134
retinopathy
    background, 24, 121
    pre-proliferative, 23, 24, 120, 121
rheumatic fever, 59, 134
rheumatoid arthritis, 3, 6, 113, 114
rheumatoid factor, 3, 113
rheumatology, 3–7, 113–14
rhinitis, allergic, 93, 151
Richter's hernia, 78, 143
rifampicin, 12, 14, 115, 116
rotator cuff tear, 87, 149
Rovsing's sign, 73, 141
rugger jersey spine, 27, 123, 124

S

salbutamol, nebulised, 10, 115
sapheno-femoral competence, 81, 145
sarcoidosis, 12, 116
scaphoid fracture, 90, 149
schistosomiasis, 51, 131
scotoma, 40, 41, 126, 127
Scottish Intercollegiate Guidelines Network (SIGN), 151
second cranial nerve, 41, 126, 127
secretin, 108, 159
seizures, 37–9, 42, 126, 127
seminoma
    diagnosis, 29, 123
    lactate dehydrogenase, 101, 155
sepsis, 103, 157
serotonin, migraine, 35, 125
seventh cranial nerve, 41, 127
Sheehan's syndrome, 24, 120
shock, haemorrhagic, 95, 153
shoulder weakness, 4, 113
sickle cell disease, 50, 130
sick sinus syndrome, 53, 133

sigmoid volvulus, 105, 159
sixth nerve palsy, 35, 125
Sjögren's syndrome, 5, 93, 113, 151
skip lesions, 63, 135, 160
sliding hernia, 106, 159
slipped upper femoral epiphysis, 89, 149
small intestine
    bacterial overgrowth, 63, 135
    distended loops, 73, 141
    elongation of villi, 63, 135
smear cells, 47, 129
smoking
    chronic obstructive pulmonary disease (COPD), 9, 115
    Crohn's disease, 63, 135
    lung cancer, 13, 116
    squamous cell carcinoma of the neck, 93, 151
sodium
    reduced plasma, 64, 136
    restricted diet, 30, 123
    restriction, alcoholic cirrhosis, 67, 136
sodium aurothiomalate, 7, 114
sodium valproate
    epilepsy, 42, 127
    side effects, 38, 126
somatostatin, increased production, 61, 135
sore throat, 91, 151
Spigelian hernia, 78, 143
spinal cord compression
    decompression, 34, 125
    symptoms, 34, 125
spinal stenosis, 7, 114
splenic abscess, 57, 134
splenomegaly, 51, 131
    causes of, 109, 159
    polycythaemia vera, 45, 129
spondylolisthesis, 7, 114
sputum staining, tuberculosis, 12, 115
squamous cell carcinoma
    lung, 13, 116
    neck, 93, 151
    oesophagus, 59, 135
stab injury, 96, 153
Staphylococcus aureus, 4, 113
    gastroenteritis, 70, 138
    infective endocarditis, 57, 134
    osteomyelitis, 87, 149
    pneumonia, 11, 14, 115, 116
    prostatitis, 155
Sternberg Reed cells, 47, 129
steroid hormones, hypopituitarism, 17, 119
steroids
    colitis, 64, 136
    Crohn's disease, 64, 136
    giant-cell arteritis, 35, 125
    inhaled, 10, 115
    long-term use, 119

steroids (continued)
    nasal spray, 93, 151
    oral, 10, 115
    ulcerative colitis, 69, 137
stools, tar-coloured, 62, 135
Streptococcus mutans, 57, 134
Streptococcus pneumoniae
    meningitis, 36, 125
    pneumonia, 10, 115
streptomycin, 12, 115
stress incontinence
    cystometrogram, 101–2, 155
    signs, 29, 123
    urodynamics, 32, 124
stroke
    aspirin, 69, 137
    investigation, 40, 126
subacromial impingement, 87, 149
subarachnoid haemorrhage, 39, 126
subdural haematoma, 39, 96, 126, 153
sulfasalazine, 7, 114
sumatriptan, headache, 125
sun ray like appearance, 87, 149
supraventricular tachycardia, 54, 133
surgery
    achalasia, 160
    colon cancer, 65, 136
    gastrointestinal, 105–10, 159–60
    indications, peptic ulcer, 109, 160
    pancreatic tumour, 23, 120
    renal cell carcinoma, 28, 32, 123, 124
    ruptured abdominal aortic aneurysm, 74, 141
surgical emergencies, 73–5, 141
swan neck deformity, 3, 113, 114
sweat test, cystic fibrosis, 10, 115
symmetrical sensory neuropathy, 23, 24, 120, 121
synacthen short test, 25, 121
syndrome of inappropriate antidiuretic hormone (SIADH), 21, 120
syringomyelia, 34, 125
systemic lupus erythematosus
    anaemia, 50, 130
    features, 6, 114
systemic sclerosis, 4, 6, 113, 114

T

tachypnoea, 63, 135
tamoxifen, 85, 147
temporal arteritis, 6, 114
temporal lobe epilepsy, 42, 127
temporal lobe lesions, 40, 127
temporal lobe seizure, 38, 126
tennis elbow, 88, 149
tension pneumothorax, 95, 153
teratoma, 29, 123
terbutaline, nebulised, 10, 115

testes
    torsion, 75, 101, 141, 155
    undescended, 101, 155
tetracosactide long test, 20, 119
tetracosactide short test, 20, 119
third nerve palsy, 35, 40, 41, 125, 127
thoracic aortic aneurysm, 79, 145
thromboangiitis obliterans, 81–2, 145
thrombophlebitis migrans, 81–2, 145
thyroglossal cyst, 91, 151
thyroid cancer, 19, 24, 119, 121
thyroid crisis, 19, 24, 119, 121
thyroid disease, 24, 120–1
thyroid hormones, hypopituitarism, 17, 119
thyroid status normalization, 19, 119
thyroid stimulating hormone receptor antibodies,
    18, 119
tics, 42–3, 127
tinnitus, 92, 151
tissue biopsy, amyloidosis, 31, 124
toes, swelling, 5, 113
tongue fasciculations, 41, 127
tonic clonic seizure, 37, 126
tonsillectomy, 91, 151
total parenteral nutrition (TPN) complications, 65, 136
transaminases, alcoholic cirrhosis, 67, 136
transient global amnesia, 39, 126
transient ischaemic attack, 39, 126
trastuzumab, 85, 147
trauma, 95–7, 153
see also fractures
tremor, benign essential, 37, 126
tricuspid regurgitation, 55, 133
trigeminal nerve, 41, 127
trigger finger, 88, 149
trochlear nerve, 41, 127
troponin, 57, 134
tuberculosis, 11, 12, 115
tubulointerstitial nephritis, 31, 124
tumour lysis syndrome, 46, 129
twelfth cranial nerve, 81, 145
typhoid, 51, 131
tyrosine kinase inhibitors, 47, 129

U

ulcerative colitis
    complications, 64, 136
    features, 63, 135
    steroids, 69, 137
ulnar nerve neuropathy, 88, 149
ultrasonography
    abdominal aortic aneurysm, 79, 145
    breast cyst, 84, 147
    cholecystitis, 68, 137
    gall bladder disease, 74, 141
    hepatocellular carcinoma, 68, 137

ultrasonography (continued)
    jaundice, 65, 107, 136, 159
    polycystic kidney disease, 28, 123
    urinary tract obstruction, 32, 101–2, 124, 155
umbilical hernia, 77, 143
undescended testes, 101, 155
unfractioned heparin, 46, 129
upper gastrointestinal disorders, 110, 160
upper gastrointestinal endoscopy
    anaemia, 63, 135
    coeliac disease, 63, 135
    gastric cancer, 62, 135
    gastrointestinal bleeding, 67, 136
    gastro-oesophageal reflux, 61, 135
urea, renal failure, 27, 123
ureteric colic, 100, 155
ureteric stone, 100, 155
urethral damage, 95, 153
urinalysis, urinary tract infection, 99, 155
urinary tract infections
    amoxicillin, 32, 124
    Escherichia coli, 30, 123
    investigation, 30, 123
    treatment, 30, 99, 123, 155
    urinalysis, 99, 155
    urine cultures, 99, 155
    urine dipstick, 101, 155
urinary tract obstruction
    renal ultrasound, 32, 124
    ultrasonography, 101–2, 155
urine cultures, urinary tract infection, 99, 155
urine dipstick, urinary tract infection, 101, 155
urine microscopy and culture, urinary tract infections,
    30, 32, 123, 124
urine osmolality, diabetes insipidus, 25, 121
urodynamic studies see cystometrogram
urology, 99–102, 155
uterine cyst, 75, 141

V

Valsalva manoeuvre, 133
varicose veins, 81, 145
vascular disorders, 81–2, 145
vascular surgery, 79–82, 145
vasculitis, 6, 114
venesection, polycythaemia vera, 45, 129
venography, deep vein thrombosis (DVT), 129
vertical nystagmus, 41, 127
vertigo, 127
vestibulocochlear nerve, 41, 127
viscus, perforated, 75, 141
vitamin B1 deficiency, 33, 41–2, 125, 127
vitamin B6 deficiency, 41–2, 127
vitamin B12
    deficiency, 49, 105, 130, 159
    replacement, 49, 130

vitamin D deficiency, 5, 113
vitamin K, 129
vomiting, Mallory Weiss tear, 62, 135

W

warfarin, 46, 129
warm antibody haemolytic anaemia,
    50, 130
Warthin's tumour, 91, 151
water deprivation test, 21, 120
Wegener's granulomatosis, 15, 117
Wenckebach's phenomenon, 53, 133
Wernicke-Korsakoff syndrome, 41–2, 127
Wilson's disease, 69, 137

X

X-ray
    appendicitis, 73, 141
    chest see chest X-ray
    kidneys, 32, 124
    kidneys, ureters and bladder see kidneys, ureters
        and bladder (KUB) X-ray
    osteoarthritis, 3, 113

Y

Yersinia enterocolitica, 70, 138

Z

Zollinger-Ellison syndrome, 110, 160